ACTA NEUROCHIRURGICA
SUPPLEMENTUM 29

Luigi Pellettieri

Surgical Versus Conservative Treatment of Intracranial Arteriovenous Malformations

A Study in Surgical Decision-Making

In collaboration with
Carl-Axel Carlsson, Sven Grevsten, Gösta Norlén,
and Christer Uhlemann

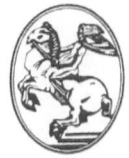

SPRINGER-VERLAG
WIEN NEW YORK

Luigi Pellettieri, M.D., Ph.D., Assistant Professor
Department of Neurosurgery, Akademiska Sjukhuset, University of
Uppsala, Sweden
Carl-Axel Carlsson, M.D., Ph.D., Assistant Professor
Department of Neurosurgery, Sahlgren Hospital, Gothenburg, Sweden
Sven Grevsten, M.D., Ph.D., Department of General Surgery,
Akademiska Sjukhuset, University of Uppsala, Sweden
Gösta Norlén, Professor in Neurosurgery, Stockholm, Sweden
Christer Uhlemann, M.D., Department of Diagnostic Radiology,
Sahlgren Hospital, Gothenburg, Sweden

With 29 Figures

Library of Congress Cataloging in Publication Data. Pellettieri, Luigi. Surgical versus conservative
treatment of intracranial arteriovenous malformations. (Acta neurochirurgica: Supplementum; 29.)
Bibliography: p. 1. Brain – Blood-vessels – Abnormalities. 2. Brain – Blood-vessels – Surgery. 3. Surgery –
Decision making. 4. Medicine – Decision making. I. Title. II. Series. III. Title: Intracranial arteriovenous malformations: a study in surgical decision-making. [DNLM: 1. Cerebral arteriovenous
malformations – Surgery. 2. Cerebral arteriovenous malformations – Therapy. 3. Probability. 4. Decision
making. 5. Prognosis. [WL355.3 P388s].

ISBN-13:978-3-211-81561-8   e-ISBN-13:978-3-7091-8567-4
DOI: 10.1007/978-3-7091-8567-4

Preface

The main aim of this study is to define the clinical criteria which must be considered in order to come to an adequate decision whether a patient with intracranial arteriovenous malformation (AVM) should be operated upon or treated conservatively. A special method was used to reduce the effects of selection. This method made it possible to evaluate the therapeutic efficacy of conservative treatment versus surgery.

The method implies that patients with equal combinations of variables (risk profiles) were compared in the two treatment lines. The variables building up the risk-profile pattern were chosen by analysing the decision process, as it was originally practiced by the surgeon who selected and treated the patients of this study. The risk profiles thus described relevant characteristics of the patient and his malformation. The variables were assigned numerical values according to their prognostic value. Summation of the variables making up the risk profile then gives each risk profile a certain value. A low value symbolizes a bad prognosis and a high value a good prognosis in both treatment groups. There were many risk profiles with the same value in both groups and a comparison could be made over a large part of the risk-profile scale. This comparison showed that surgical treatment of AVM can always be justified, although the indications for surgery are less strong in patients with low risk-profile values. The outcome for patients in this part of the risk-profiles scale seems to be independent of the method of treatment. The method of assessment described above can be used in clinical practice for each individual patient with AVM. Each patients risk-profile value gives an indication of the prognosis for surgical and conservative treatment. The method described may be used for prognostic evaluation of alternative treatment lines also in other diseases.

I would like to express my gratitude to the Universities of Gothenburg and Uppsala for their financial support, which made it possible for me to accomplish this study.

Uppsala, December 1979

LUIGI PELLETTIERI

Contents

I. General Introduction

Although a large number of reports on arteriovenous malformations (AVM) have been published since the latter half of the nineteenth century (see review articles [10, 21, 29, 33, 38, 40, 48]), the criteria for selection of an adequate mode of therapy for patients with AVM are still the subject of controversy.

A number of patho-anatomical studies have been carried out in endeavour to establish the pathogenesis and develop a system of classification as a basis for clinical decision-making [5, 7, 8, 15, 25, 27, 32, 34, 44, 53]. With the introduction of cerebral angiography it became possible to map out the functional architecture of AVM (size, position, vascularization). This was a prerequisite for surgical treatment. The first reports on surgical treatment of AVM appeared in the nineteenthirties [5, 6] and the first principles for surgical treatment of these malformations were then formulated [1, 6]. These principles were in line with those applied at that time for tumour surgery. Only small AVM, situated in areas of minor importance, were considered operable. Advances in surgical techniques and methods of anaesthesia during the subsequent decades have meant that increasingly large and increasingly many AVM have become operable. Parallel with this broadening of the indications for operation, however, the criteria for surgical treatment have been called in question and the still unresolved controversy concerning surgery contra conservative treatment has grown up. Several studies of series of operated and nonoperated patients [9, 17, 28, 31, 33, 35, 37, 40, 50] have been published, without showing unequivocally which is the right treatment policy. In addition to these two alternatives, a third possibility has arisen in recent years: elimination of the malformation by nonclassical surgical methods, such as X-ray irradiation [14, 42, 49], stereotactic cryosurgery [56], embolization [22] and catheterization for occlusion by means of a balloon [46]. The value of these methods and possibilities for further development have not yet been exhaustively explored. These methods will therefore not be discussed in this study. The aim of the study is to compare the therapeutic efficacy of conservative treatment and surgery (total extirpation) in comparable patient-AVM constellations and formulate principles for selection of treatment.

The clinician's dilemma when confronted with a patient with AVM has been formulated by Pia [39], in his introduction to the Giessen symposium on cerebral angioma in 1974, as follows: "In the absence of an absolute rule to guide his decision, the surgeon must carefully plot each borderline case against the abscissa of danger and the ordinate of benefit." When treating a patient with AVM, however, the clinician has no clear guidelines to follow. Indead, one has the impression at times that two diametrically opposed lines of action may lead to the same ultimate result. The clinical studies in series of operated and/or nonoperated patients that have been published during the last few decades have admittedly led to an increased knowledge of the disease as such but have not really made the decision process for or against surgery any easier. In a complicated situation in which it is not possible to analyse the finer points and there are no firm rules to follow, it is perhaps natural that summary policies are preferred. While it is true that adoption of an extreme policy facilitates the decision process, however, it may easily lead to a less than optimal decision. Two contrasting and simple treatment approaches have polarized more and more during the last few decades: one group advocates an aggressive surgical policy towards AVM, while the other argues in favour of a purely conservative treatment policy.

The basic principles for surgical treatment with total extirpation as the objective were laid down by Cushing and Bailey in the USA and Olivecrona in Europe during the thirties. Tönnis [53], Krayenbühl [18], McKissock [26], Norlén [28], and Krenchel [19] developed the surgical technique during the forties and fifties and Kunc [20], Sano [45], Buche [2], Walter and Bischof [57], Pia [39] and Yaşargil [59] and others have since made further contributions to the surgical management of AVM.

Support for the conservative approach has arisen from the disappointments and failures that have unquestionably occurred as a result of an over-enthusiastic adherence to the surgical policy. Troupp [52] has been one of the main champions of the conservative approach. It might be claimed that the neurosurgeons who use forms of treatment other than total extirpation, such as embolization, irradiation etc., have also in a sense rejected the energetic surgical approach.

It is tempting to argue that the "correct" line of action lies somewhere between these two extreme approaches, *i.e*, that the situation must be judged "from case to case". But to make this claim without laying down detailed guidelines for action in each specific case is merely to argue that there is an adequate approach, without saying what that approach is.

Many people who have endeavoured to judge patients "from case to case" have probably felt the want of adequate criteria upon which to base the decision. The choice in such situation may easily be instinctive: the importance attached to different factors differs according to the surgical skill and previous experience of the person taking the decision. For example, some people attach great importance to the size of the malformation and this variable alone may be decisive for their subsequent line of action. In a similar way, too much importance may be attached to the position of the malformation, its vascularization, measured in terms of the number of feeding arteries, or the symptoms at onset (haemorrhage or epilepsy) when deciding between surgical and conservative treatment.

There is no doubt that many variables must be weighed against each other when deciding whether or not to operate. Several studies in different contexts have shown that human beings have a limited capacity to evaluate information for decision-making purposes [30]. It has been found that, above a certain level, access to increased information does not result in better decisions, even though the decision-maker may be convinced that it does. When faced with the problem of reaching a decision as to which treatment policy to adopt in patients with AVM, people often try to obtain more information in endeavour to increase the chances of making the right decision. This often means that they are unable to handle all the information they have available and are forced to give priority to certain parts of the information in order to obtain a reasonable basis for the decision. Since it has been shown that people tend to choose information which supports their own hypotheses and neglect information which does not, such factors in the decision process have an obvious influence on the subsequent treatment.

Aim of the Study

This study has mainly been prompted by the uncertainty and lack of clear guidelines for treatment of AVM. The main aim was therefore *to define the clinical criteria which must always be considered in order to reach an adequate decision as to whether a patient with AVM should be operated upon or given conservative treatment.*

This presupposes

1. that the AVM-patient variables that are of prognostic importance can be identified;

2. that these variables can be graded and weighed against each other;

3. that this "weighing of variables" makes it possible to construct a "risk profile" for each individual patient;

4. that these "risk profiles" can be quantified; and

5. that equivalent or similar risk profiles are found among operated and nonoperated patients. This means that equivalent or similar risk profiles in the two groups can be compared despite the fact that the operated and nonoperated groups differ as a whole, owing to the clinician's original selection.

Methodological Considerations

The study comprises a series of operated and nonoperated patients with AVM, according to McCormick's [25] classification. Venous angioma, cavernoma, teleangiectasia and varix have thus not been studied.

A problem when comparing the prognosis between operated and nonoperated groups of patients in many previous studies has been that there have been obvious differences between the groups, owing to selection, so that they have not been directly comparable. In the present retrospective analysis this source of error has been avoided. Instead of comparing the mortality and morbidity in the groups as a whole, the prognosis has been correlated to different patient and AVM variables ("risk profiles"). By rating the importance of the variables according to the results, a quantitative risk profile can be constructed for each patient. This means that the prognosis for patients with equivalent risk profiles can be compared in the operated and the nonoperated group despite the fact that the groups as a whole are not comparable.

In order to carry out this programme, it seemed natural to describe the anatomy of the AVM in Chapter II as it appeared from the X-ray investigations in our patients. Thus, the appearance, size, position and vascularization of the malformations are described. These data are analysed in relation to the patient's sex and age. This static description of the material is supplemented in Chapter III by the clinician's integrated impression of the dynamic course, which forms the basis of his selection of patients for operation or conservative treatment. By analysing the clinician's management of the case, the patient-AVM variables which governed his decision can be identified. This line of reasoning has been carried out *"per absurdum"*: it has been hypothesized that the patient selection was correct, and the patients who were operated upon have been regarded as operable and those not operated upon as inoperable. Variables of importance for the decision process have then been included in the risk profiles which have been used for the subsequent analyses. In Chapter IV (nonoperated patients) and Chapter V (operated patients) equivalent risk profiles are challenged with the long-term results.

This makes it possible to determine whether one or other method of treatment has a favourable or unfavourable influence on equivalent risk profiles. It is of subordinate importance in this context whether or not the original selection was correct. In fact, some inconsistency in the original decision process is a prerequisite for the study, since it is based on finding equivalent risk profiles in both groups. In Chapter VI all the risk profiles have been quantified symbolically so that their prognostic significance can be measured. This means that the probable consequences of a decision for or against surgery can be predicted for each risk profile.

II. Morphological Aspects

Luigi Pellettieri and Christer Uhlemann *

Introduction

In the previous chapter the overall aims of the study were formulated. The purpose of the study is to analyse retrospectively a
clinical series of patients with AVM and define adequate criteria for
selection of the most suitable mode of therapy—surgery or conservative treatment. A prerequisite for the study was that comparisons of
the results of treatment in the two groups were made between patients
who were comparable with respect to individual characteristics as
well as variables relating to AVM. This chapter presents an analysis
of the clinical material with respect to AVM vascularization, size and
location. These variables are related to each other and to the patient's
age and sex. This description of the static part of the patient-AVM
constellation constitutes a basis for subsequent analysis.

Classification

Virchow [55] was the first worker in modern times to describe angiomatous intracranial malformations, as long ago as in the mid-
nineteenth century. In 1928 Dandy [6] and Cushing and Bailey [5]
presented small series of arteriovenous "aneurysms" in the brain. In
the same year the latter authors proposed the following classification
of intracranial angiomatous malformations: a) teleangiectasia,
b) venous angioma and c) arterial (arteriovenous) angioma. They
differentiated these malformations from haemangioblastoma on the
basis that the latter tumour lacked nervous tissue interposed between
the angiomatous structures. Russel and Rubinstein [44] reported in 1971
that the stroma in cavernous angioma was sometimes completely
lacking in nervous tissue and they included this type of malformation in the above classification. A similar classification

---

* Department of Diagnostic Radiology, Sahlgren Hospital, University of
Gothenburg, Gothenburg, Sweden.

was proposed by McCormick[25] in 1966, except that he included venous varices as a subgroup to venous angiomas. Some authors, for example Hamby[11] and Potter[42], challenge the above classification and consider that all, or at least the overwhelming majority, of the tumours described above should in fact be classified as arteriovenous malformations. Hamby[11] stated in 1957 that Olivecrona and Riives agreed with Cushing and Bailey that these vascular malformations were impossible to differentiate histologically and that the difference was physiological and depended on the degree of arterialization of the lesion. He also stated that little, if any, evidence in support of the occurrence of pure venous malformations has been presented since the introduction of angiography. According to Hamby[11] the cases in which the possibility of venous angioma remains are patients who have sustained intracerebral haemorrhage and in whom very small conglomerates of tortuous veins are found at operation. He refers, however, to a report by Dorothy Russell (1954) in which she describes a relatively well-preserved preparation of this type which was found on histological examination to contain vessels with lamina elastica of the type that is typical for arteries. Potter[42] goes so far as to state that practically all angiomatous malformations are in fact arteriovenous at some level.

Most authors, e.g., McCormick[25], consider, however, that angiomatous malformations can be divided into the following types: a) capillary telangiectasia, b) cavernous angioma, c) AV malformations and d) venous malformations.

This study deals with *arteriovenous malformations* (AVM). In the Anglo-Saxon literature the synonymous term "AV angiomas" is used about equally often. The fundamental point in the diagnosis of this lesion is the angiographically demonstrable shunt. AVM is the commonest and most thoroughly described vascular malformation of the CNS and accounts, in different material, for between 1.5 and 4% of verified intracranial expansive processes.

Macroscopically, an AVM consists of a tortuous conglomerate of veins and arteries which are abnormal in both length and calibre. This bundle of vessels makes up the actual malformation and replaces the normal capillary bed of the region concerned. Kaplan[15] considered the lesion to be a vestigial primitive arteriovenous communication which would normally have been replaced by a capillary network. It is thus a congenital anomaly, which may grow and destroy the brain tissue but which does not exhibit cell proliferation. Several authors have discussed the growth tendency of AVM. For example, Höök[13], in an angiographic study of nonoperated AVM patients, found growth in 8 out of 13. Waltimo[58] found growth in 12 out

of 21 nonoperated AVM patients studied by angiography, whereas
the size of the AVM was unchanged in 8 and one AVM had decreased
in size.

The arteries are usually dilated, tortuous and longer than normal
and the veins are proportionately even more dilated, sometimes
aneurysmal. AVM occurs in all sizes, from microscopic (or at least
subangiographic) to large malformations engaging entire lobes of the
brain. The adjacent brain tissue is often atrophic and a more
generalized atrophy may also occur, probably owing to the steal
phenomenon.

The microscopical appearance of the malformations is variable
and complex. Well-defined arteries and veins may be seen alternating
with less well-differentiated vascular structures. Degenerative changes
in the form of hyalinized vessels, fibrosis, atheromatosis in arteries
and thrombi in veins, as well as necrosis after repeated minor haemorrhages, are common.

Patients and Methods

The study comprises 166 consecutive patients with intracranial
AVM who were investigated and treated at the Department of
Neurosurgery at Sahlgren Hospital in Gothenburg between 1953 and
1971. The study thus covers an 18-year period. All AVM were
demonstrated by angiography (in many cases supplemented with
encephalography and/or ventriculography). Purely dural AVM are
not included in this study.

The coarse anatomy of all 166 AVM could be described from the
combined information obtained from radiological reports, available
X-ray films and operation reports. This description comprises the
location and size of the AVM, as well as its vascularization and
draining venous sinuses.

AVM situated adjacent to the fissures of Sylvius and Rolando or
in the posterior fossa have been combined as belonging to nonsilent
areas, while other locations have been considered to be silent areas.
In the frontal projection the location has been divided into two
groups: superficially situated AVM (cortical and subcortical) and
deeply situated AVM (in or close to the midline). In the frontal
projection a curved line from the sagittal sinus through the internal
capsule to the base of the skull refines the borderline between deeply
and superficially situated AVM (see Fig. 23, Chapter IV). Ventricular
and paraventricular AVM have of course been classified as deep.
Note, however, that an AVM on the medial side of the hemisphere
has been classified as being deeply situated despite the fact that
anatomically it may be regarded as cortical or subcortical. In border-

line cases AVM were grouped as deep or superficial, with reference to the location of the main part of the malformation.

When classifying AVM according to size, the malformations have been broadly divided into small and large AVM. The dividing line between small and large malformations has been arbitrarily set at 3 cm in diameter. In view of the sometimes irregular shape of the malformations and the varying magnification in the films, the diameter used has been the maximum diameter. Note that the size has been assessed in relation to the malformed vascular bundle which constitutes the actual shunt, although large venous channels are at times the most conspicuous structure.

The vascularization of the AVM has not been used as a variable in subsequent parts of the study since it is not expressly stated as a motive for or against operation by the clinician (see Chapter III). It may be assumed, however, that the vascularization is directly related to the size and location of the AVM, which have been used in the original decision process. Thus, when judging the operability in terms of the size and location of the AVM, the clinician may include the complexity of the vascularization as a secondary factor even though this is not usually stated in the case records.

When analysing the coarse anatomy of the total material, the arterial vascularization is stated in relation to the main branches, i.e., the anterior cerebral artery, middle cerebral artery, posterior cerebral artery, external carotid artery and vertebral artery. The venous drainage is stated in relation to the large sinus draining the malformation.

A detailed radiological survey could be carried out for 88 of the 166 patients. These selected films have been used to study the terminal branches of the arteries supplying the AVM and also to study the draining veins. "Terminal branches" in this context means branches which supply the malformation and must be ligated at operation. The number of terminal branches has been related to the size and location of the AVM. Only those AVM in which the number of terminal branches could be counted with certainty have been included. These cases have been divided into four groups, depending on whether the AVM was supplied by one, two, three or more than three terminal arteries. The relationship between the number of terminal branches and location of the AVM in silent or nonsilent areas could be analysed in 61 cases. The relationship between the number of terminal branches and location of the AVM in superficial or deep zones could be analysed in 41 cases.

The venous drainage could be analysed in 59 cases. Special efforts have been made to correlate different types of venous drainage with the occurrence of haemorrhage.

Results

*Position and Size of the AVM in Relation to the Patient's Age
and Sex*

AVM occurs about equally often in the right and left hemisphere
(43% right, 42% left). There is a certain left predominance, however, for the fissure of Sylvius and the motor region (54% left,

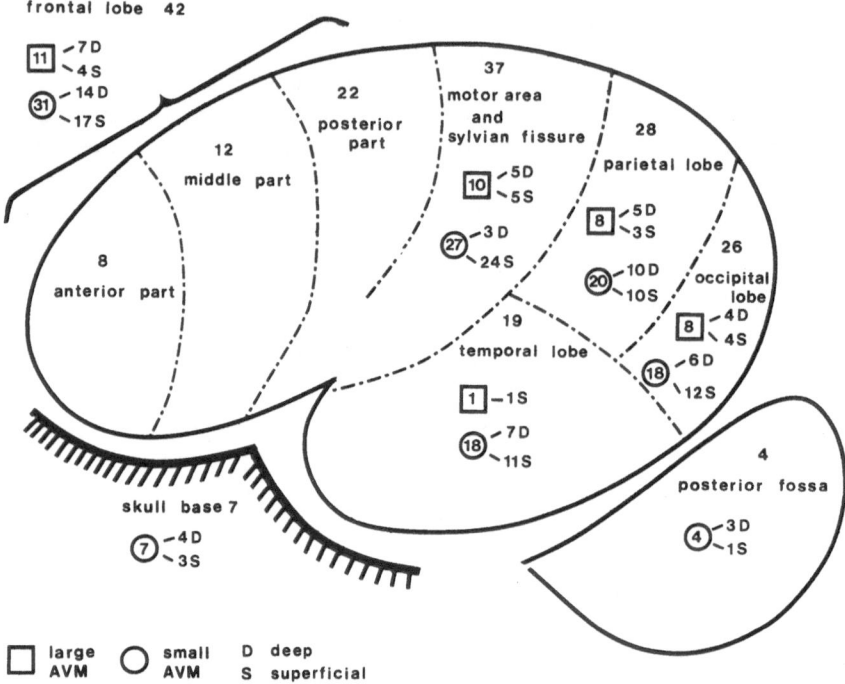

Fig. 1. Distribution of large/small AVM and deep/superficial AVM in different
brain areas

46% right). In women, the lesion occurs more often in the left hemisphere (53% left, 41% right), whereas the situation is the opposite in
men (45% right, 35% left). AVM in the motor region and fissure
of Sylvius occurs somewhat more often in men than in women.
Altogether 116 AVM (70%) were situated in silent areas and 50
(30%) in nonsilent areas. Fig. 1 shows the distribution of AVM by
lobe, and the deep/superficial distribution is shown in Table 1. Three
intraventricular AVM are not included in the distribution by lobe.
Two of them were large AVM and one was small.

Table 1. *Deeply and Superficially Located AVM Versus AVM-Size*

	Number of patients	Small AVM	Large AVM
Deep AVM	71	48	23
Superficial AVM	95	78	17
Total	166	126	40

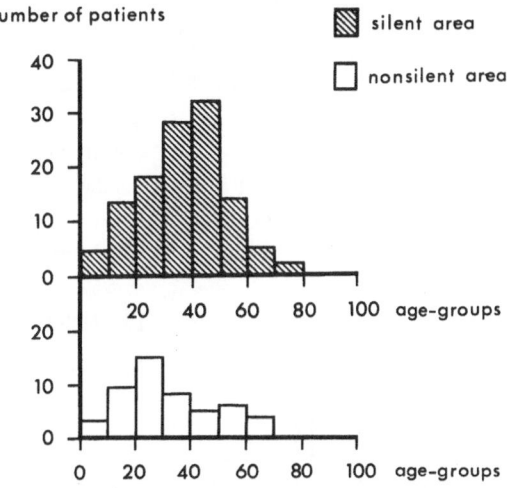

Fig. 2. Distribution of AVM in "silent" and "nonsilent" areas, versus age

Fig. 2 shows the patients' ages in relation to the distribution of AVM in silent and nonsilent areas. AVM giving symptoms before the age of 30 years are more often situated in nonsilent areas, while those giving symptoms after the age of 30 years are usually situated in silent areas.

When classifying the AVM by size, 126 (76%) were classed as small and 40 (24%) as large. The distribution of large and small AVM by lobe and their distribution in the frontal plane is shown in Fig. 1 and Table 1, respectively. The relationship between AVM size and the patient's age is shown in Fig. 3. The ratio of small to large AVM is significantly higher in the 10–50 years age-group than in the 50–90 years group. After the age of 40 years large AVM are more common in silent than in nonsilent areas (Fig. 4). The distribution of large and small AVM in men and women is approximately the same (76% small and 24% large in men, compared to 70% and 30% respectively, in women).

number of AVM

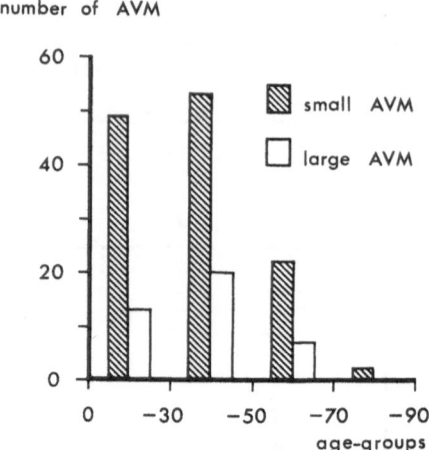

Fig. 3. Distribution of small and large AVM, versus age

number of patients

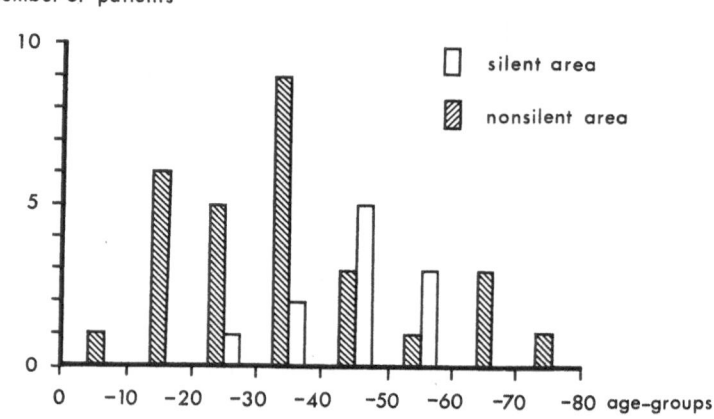

Fig. 4. Distribution of large AVM in "silent" and "nonsilent" areas, versus age

Arterial Vascularization of AVM

Main branches: The arterial vascularization was unilateral or bilateral. Bilateral vascularization was mainly found in deeply situated AVM. Fig. 5 shows how often large arteries were engaged in AVM. Note that the incidence figure for the external carotid artery is too low as selective angiography of this artery was caried out in only a few cases. Fortyeight AVM were supplied by two or more of the large cerebral vessels, in different combinations. The combination anterior cerebral artery + middle cerebral artery occurred 18 times; middle cerebral artery + posterior cerebral artery 14 times; anterior cerebral artery + posterior cerebral artery 6 times; anterior cerebral artery + middle cerebral artery + posterior cerebral artery 10 times. Combinations with branches of the external carotid artery are not presented owing to the uncertainty described above.

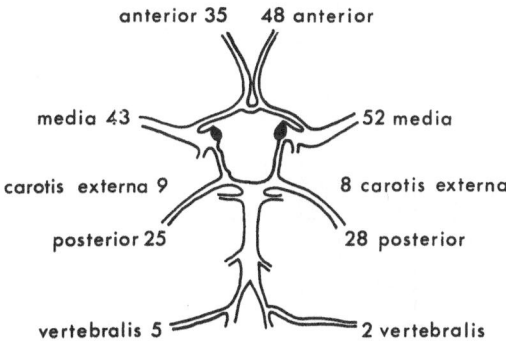

Fig. 5. Arterial supply to AVM, main branches only

Arterial aneurysms were observed in combination with AVM in 4 patients: 2 men and 2 women. One of these patients had 2 arterial aneurysms. Three of the aneurysms were situated in the artery supplying the AVM, whereas the other two were situated in other arteries.

Vasospasm was observed in only two out of the 166 cases.

Terminal branches: The arterial vascularization of the AVM could be studied in detail in a subgroup. Fig. 6 and 7 show the relationship between the number of terminal branches and the location of the malformation. This comparison reveals no difference in the number of terminal branches between AVM situated in silent and nonsilent areas. Deeply situated AVM seem, however, to be supplied by two or more terminal branches somewhat more often than superficially situated AVM.

The relationship between the number of terminal branches and size of the AVM is shown in Fig. 8. Small malformations were usually supplied by few terminal branches, whereas large malformations tended to be supplied by more branches, usually more than three.

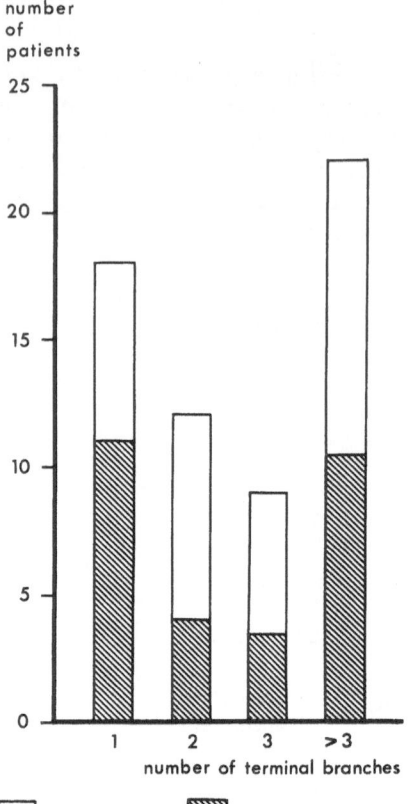

Fig. 6. Distribution of AVM in "silent" and "nonsilent" areas, versus number of terminal branches

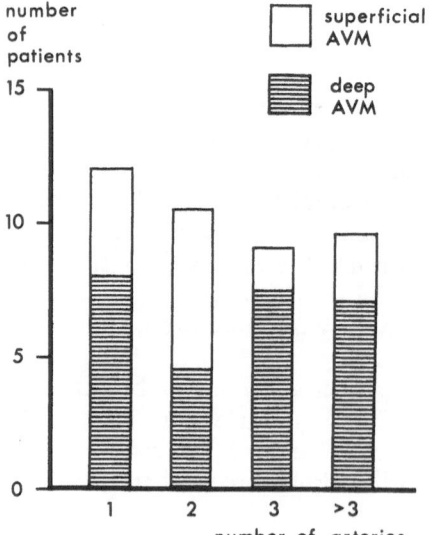

Fig. 7. Distribution of superficial and deep AVM, versus number of terminal branches

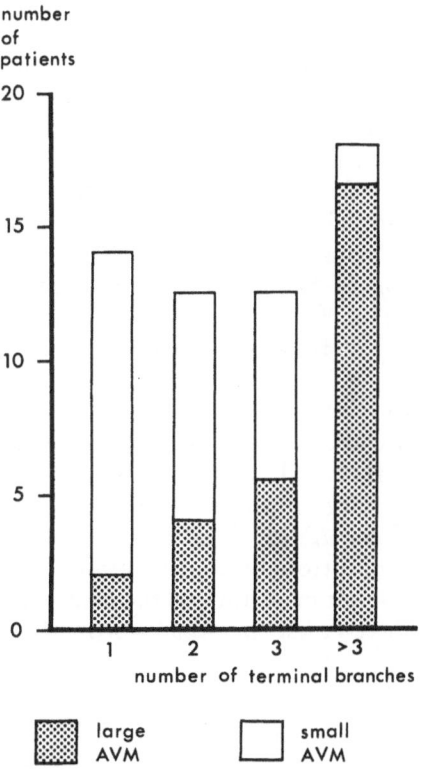

Fig. 8. Relationship between the number of terminal branches and the size
of the AVM

Venous Drainage of AVM

Venous sinuses: The sagittal sinus was the draining sinus
114 times. Drainage into other sinuses was less common (Fig. 9). As
the figure shows, venous drainage into more than one sinus was found
in certain cases.

Draining veins: When analysing the assessable angiographic
material with respect to venous drainage from AVM we were struck
by the frequently extraordinary course of the bloodstream. One
would expect an AVM to be supplied by branches from adjacent large
arteries and drained by veins normally occurring in the area in their
normal direction of flow. In most cases the bloodstream (*i.e.*, the
angiographically demonstrated flow of contrast medium) showed the

physiological direction, in familiar venous structures, although they
were sometimes tortuous and dilated. Deviations from the normal
drainage were sometimes observed, however. These deviations were
related to reversal of flow in draining veins.

In addition to taking the expected paths, the venous drainage
sometimes occurred partly against the direction of flow, *i.e.*, the blood
(contrast medium) backed out into veins which normally drain into
the natural drainage vein. For example, retrograde flow sometimes
occurred in central veins or sinuses. There were also cases in which
the normal direction of flow of the vein(s) was not known but in
which the direction of flow was reversed after extirpation of the
AVM. The direction of flow seen postoperatively may be assumed to
be physiological.

Another pattern of venous drainage was observed mainly in connection with superficial convexity veins. In some patients the contrast
medium ran out in several, often superficial, veins, which either
anastomosed with a large drainage vein or were situated in the immediate vicinity of the AVM. This occurred with a distinctly slow
flow-rate, contrasting strongly to the rapid flow usually seen in
drainage vessels. The ultimate fate of the contrast medium could not
be ascertained in these cases. In other words, the flow could not be

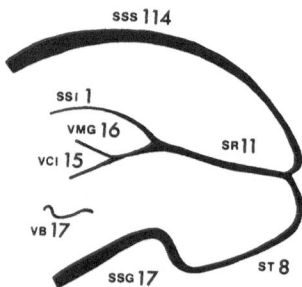

Fig. 9. Frequency of AVM drainage via different sinuses: *SSS* sinus sagittalis
superior, *SSI* sinus sagittalis inferior, *SR* sinus rectus, *VCI* vena cerebri interna,
VMG vena Magna Galeni, *VB* vena basalis, *SSG* sinus sigmoideus, *ST* sinus trans-
versus

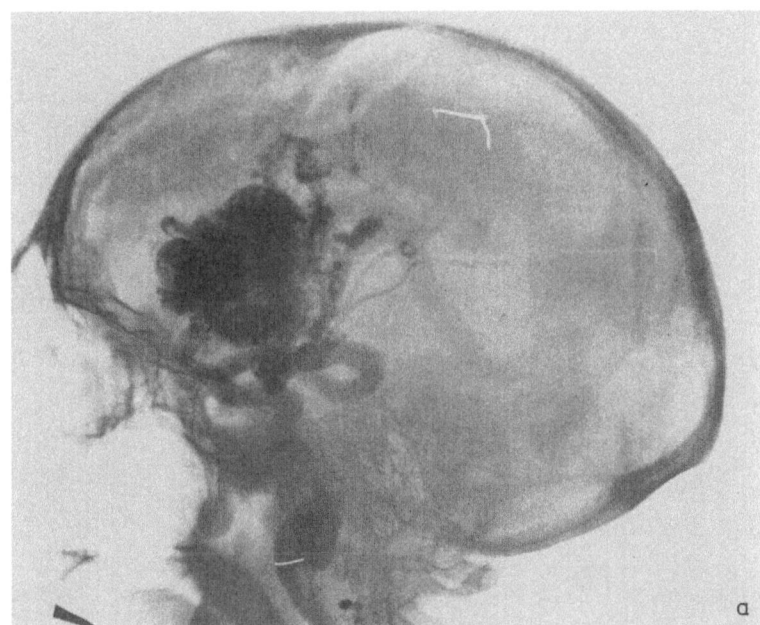

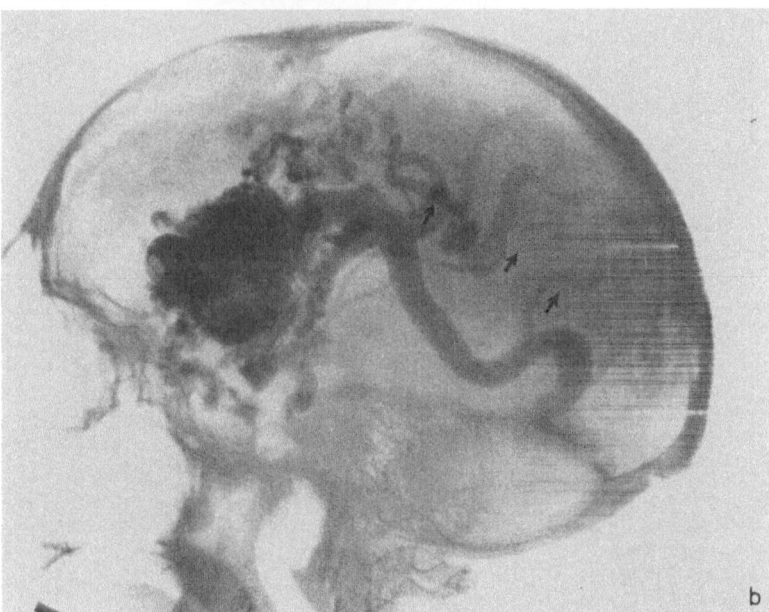

Fig. 10. AVM showing backflow in superficial veins from the main draining vein: 38 year-old man presenting with grand mal seizures. There is a leftsided AVM located basally, deeply within the frontal lobe with arterial supply from both sides. The main draining vein is a dilated vein of Labbé. The contrast medium can be seen passing out in its tributaries where the direction of flow is contrary to the anticipated. Arrows indicate the direction of bloodflow (10 a, 10 b)

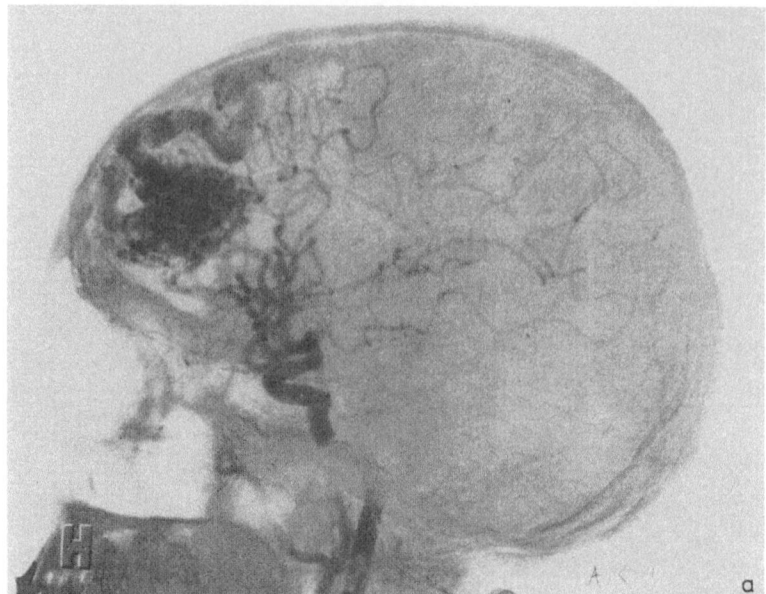

Fig. 11 a

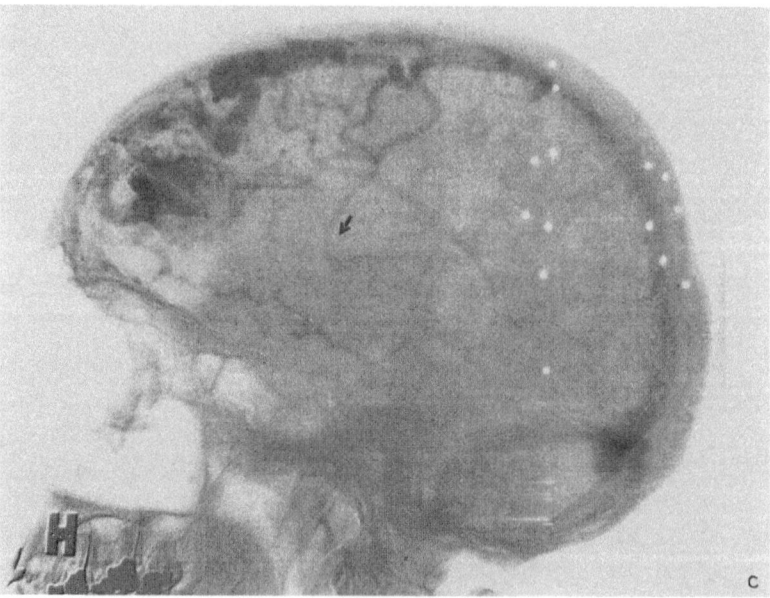

Fig. 11 c

Fig. 11. AVM showing reversal of flow in draining vein after surgical removal
of the lesion: Male, 26 years old, with epileptic seizures. Angiography shows a
rightsided, deeply located frontal AVM where the main venous drainage occurs
through a tortuous, medially located vein to the sagittal sinus. There is backflow

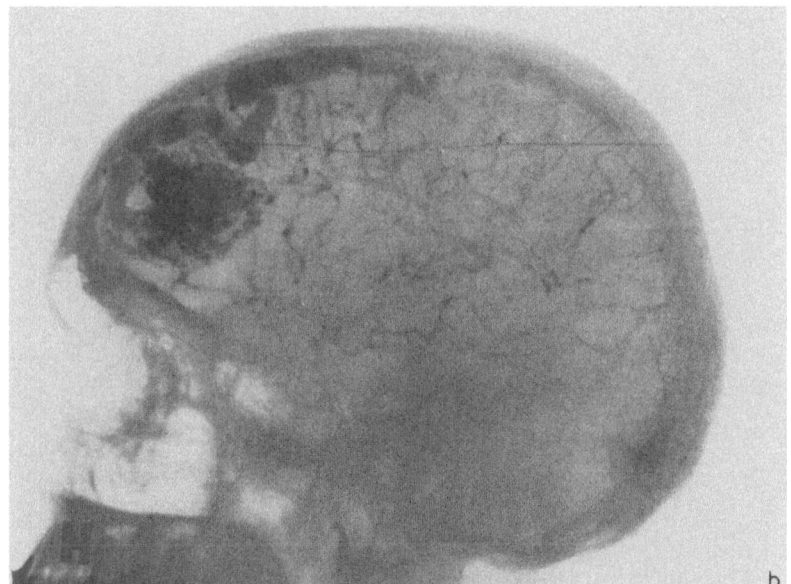

Fig. 11 b

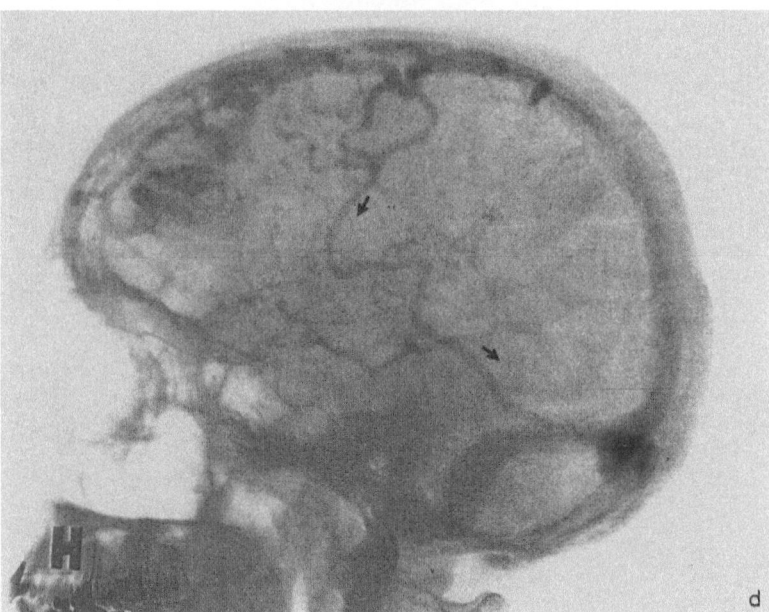

Fig. 11 d

through a superficial anastomotic vein from the sagittal sinus to the sigmoid sinus (the vein of Trolard and the vein of Labbé respectively). After surgical removal of the AVM the direction of flow in the vein of Trolard is reversed and now physiological. Arrows indicate the direction of blood-flow (Figs. a—d preop., e—h postop.)

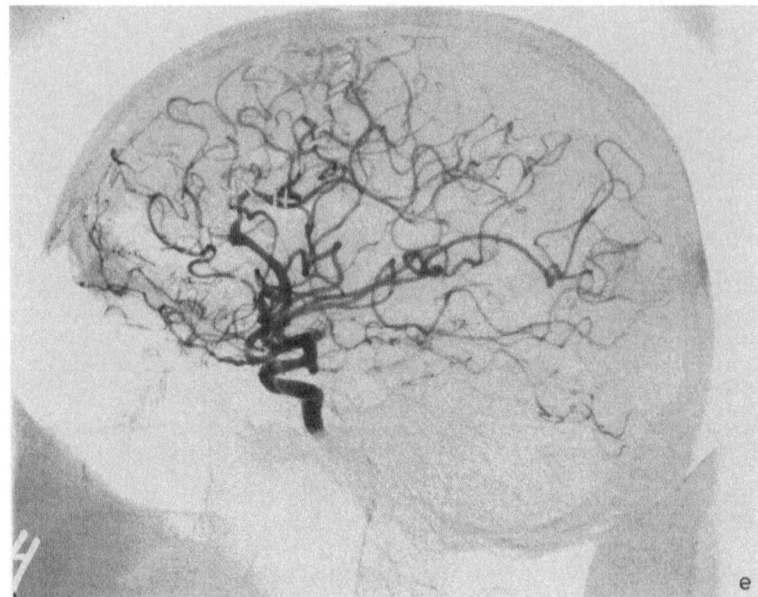

Fig. 11 e

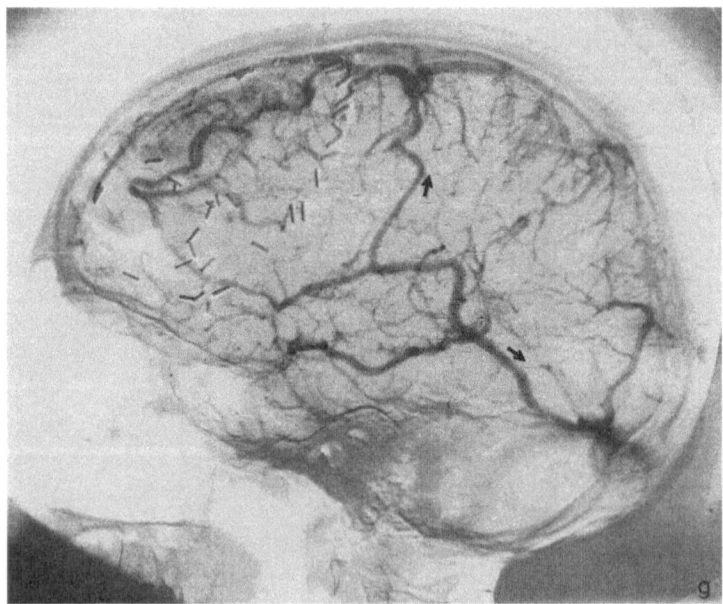

Fig. 11 g

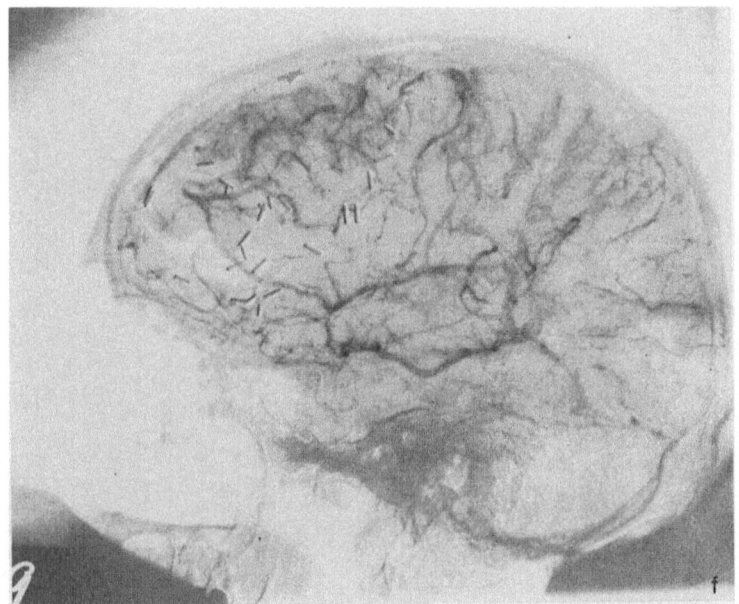

Fig. 11 f

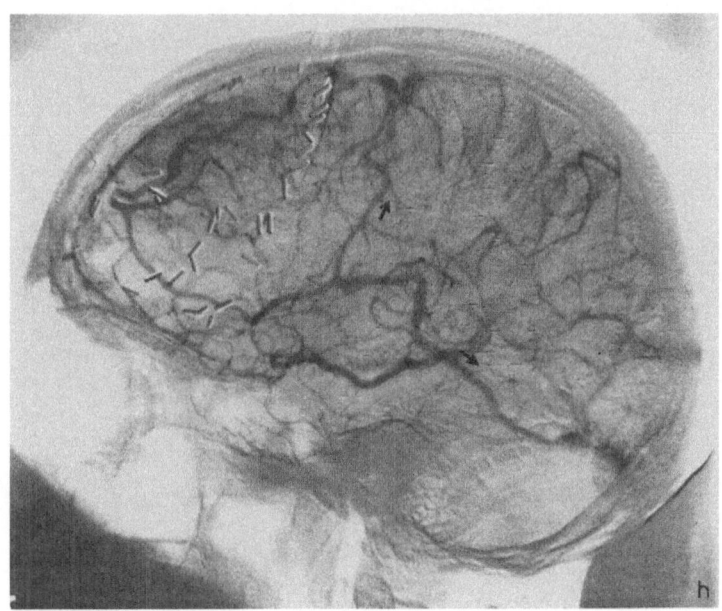

Fig. 11 h

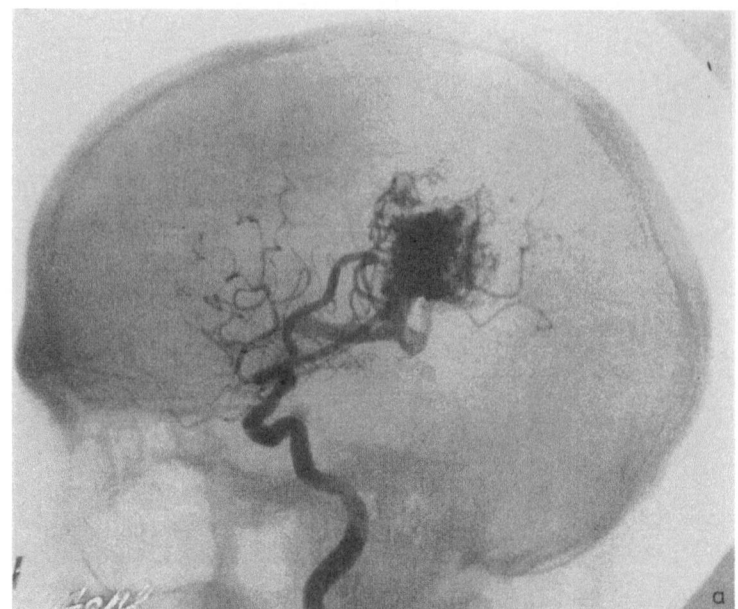

Fig. 12 a

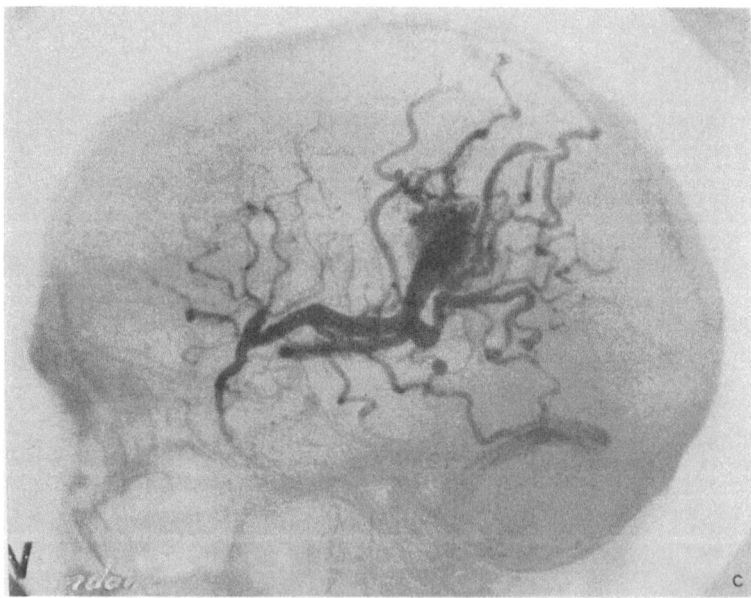

Fig. 12 c

Fig. 12. AVM showing massive backflow in superficial convexity veins: Male
patient, 62 years of age with epileptic seizures 1941, −42 and −50. 1965 intracerebral haemorrhage preceding the angiography. There is a wedge-shaped AVM
with partly deep venous drainage but above all superficial drainage to a wide

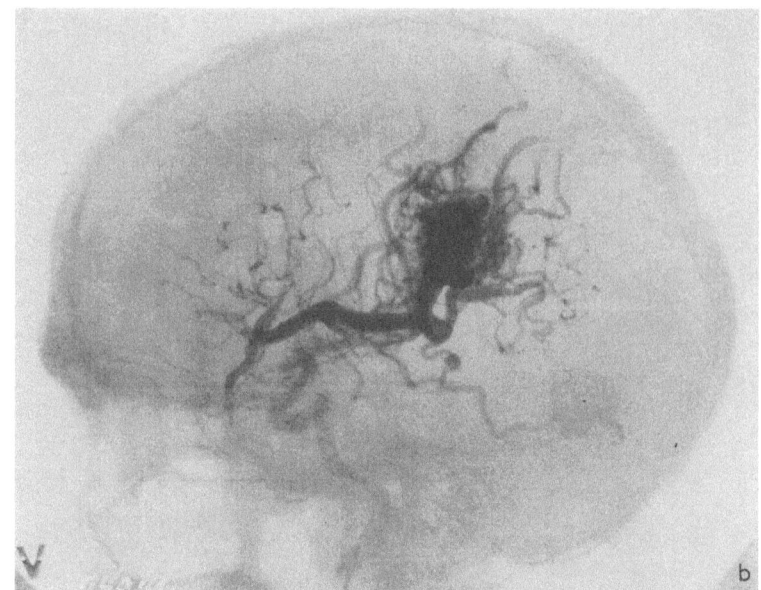

Fig. 12 b

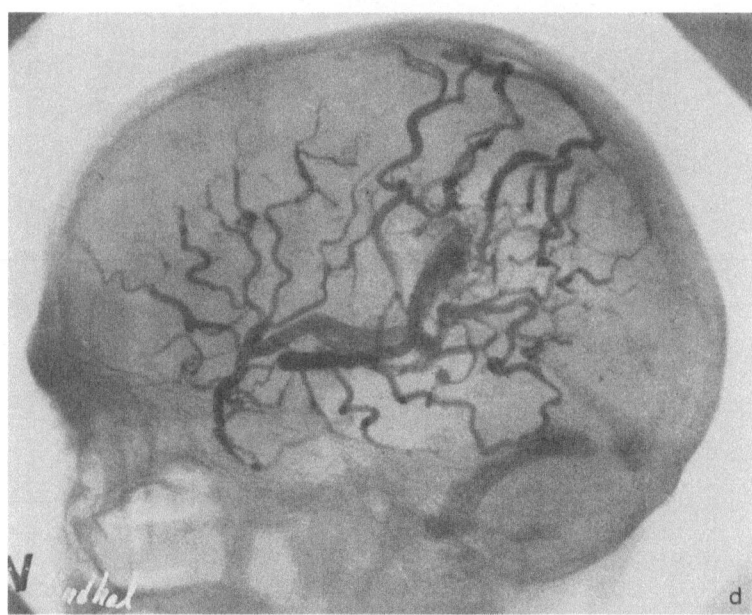

Fig. 12 d

superficial middle cerebral vein from which a large number of superficial veins are seen contrast-filled. Most of these veins terminate in the superior sagittal sinus but there is a definite reversal of flow in these veins in the vicinity of the middle cerebral vein (Figs. a, b, c, d, e, f, g)

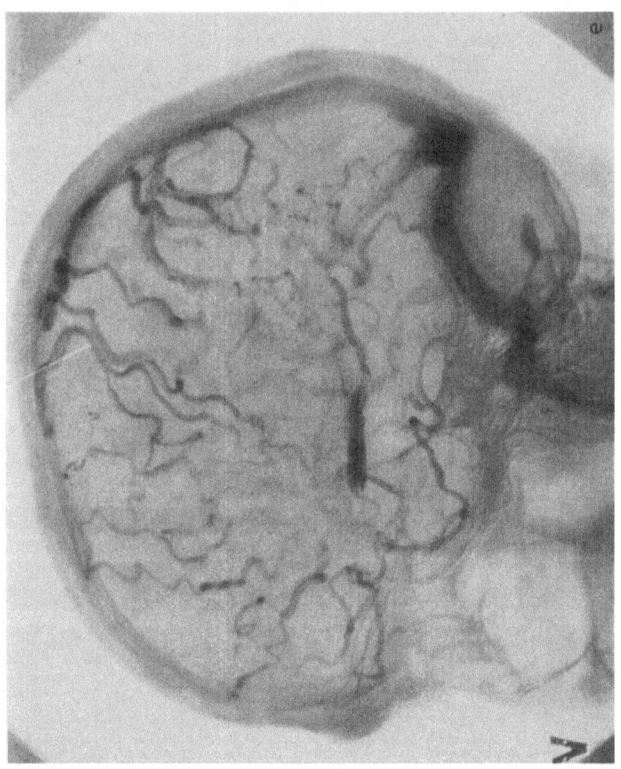

Fig. 12 e

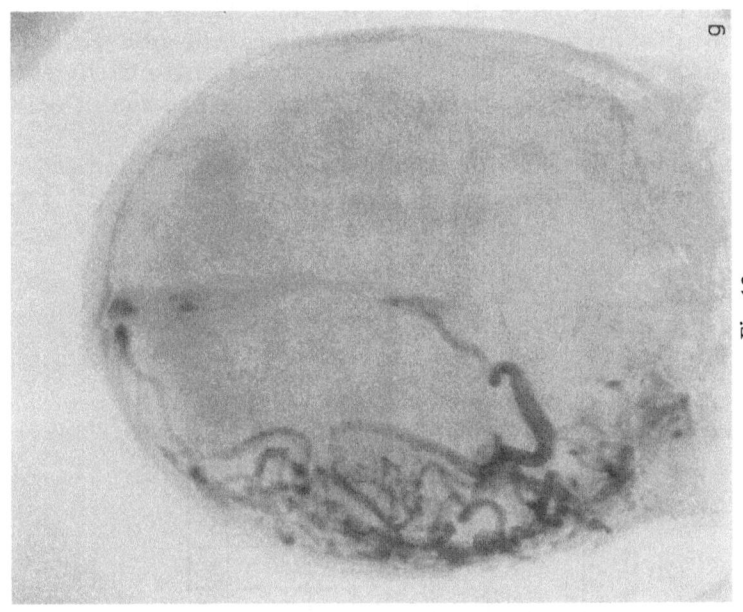

Fig. 12 g

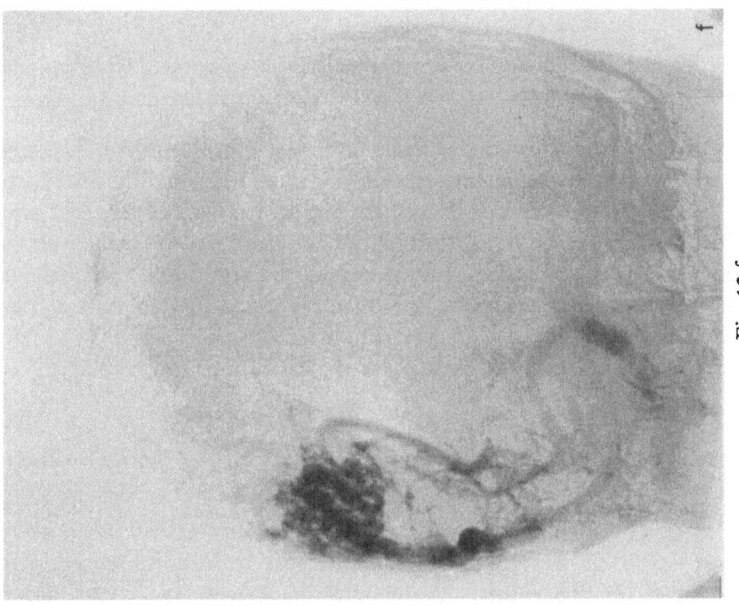

Fig. 12 f

followed to any of the sinuses and successive dilution of the contrast medium occurred during the series of films. Once again, it may be assumed that the veins concerned are recipients of an overflow from the main drainage vein. It is possible that these cases merely represent inadequate angiographic technique and that the situation is the equivalent of the backflow described above.

Occasional patients exhibited anomalous venous drainage in that one or more of the draining veins had a distinctly bizarre appearance,

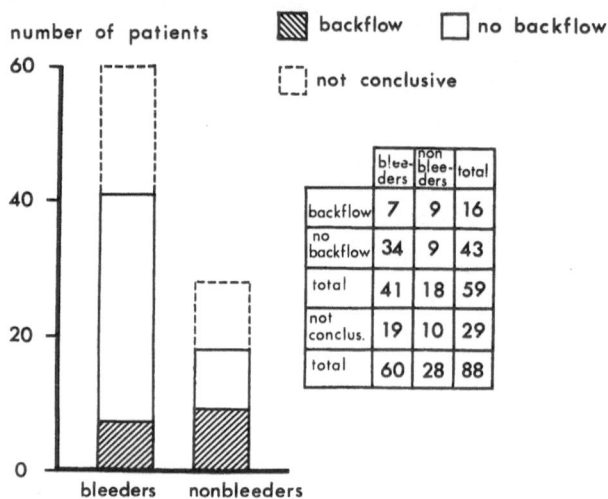

Fig. 13. Relationship between angiographically demonstrated backflow and haemorrhage

with a highly tortuous course and relatively small calibre. These veins sometimes drained into a larger vein or sinus at a considerable distance from the AVM and in conflict with the normal drainage paths. The most likely explanation is that these were aberrant veins related to the patient's malformation, but it cannot be ruled out that this group includes exceptional cases representing a backflow of the type discussed above.

Examples of reversal of flow in draining veins are given in Figs. 10, 11, and 12.

Relationship Between AVM With Aberrant Venous Drainage and Haemorrhage

It might be speculated that backflow in veins, as discussed above, is an expression of a circulatory adaptation to the increased volume load caused by the shunt. Veins with backflow might act as a sort of safey-valve, leading to a reduction of the total intravascular pressure. This mechanism might be related to haemorrhage. Reports of haemorrhage at onset have been related to the occurrence of backflow in veins as defined above. Backflow could only be studied in 59 patients as study of this phenomenon presupposes an acceptable angiographic examination. Backflow was found in 7 out of 41 (17.0%) patients with haemorrhage and in 9 out of 18 (50.0%) without haemorrhage (Fig. 13).

Discussion

In the strict and normal sense, "operability" means that a lesion is technically amenable for operation. However, the concept also includes an assessment of the risks of the procedure in relation to the patient's age and condition. In the case of patients with AVM, the potential risk of fatal or disabling haemorrhage must also be considered. This calculation of risk adds a new dimension to the assessment. The operable/inoperable concept is still valid but a new factor is added: the indications for operation. Depending on how the clinician views the risks, the indications for operation are broadened or restricted.

The number of terminal arterial branches has not been used as a variable for decision-making in this study. However, there is a clear relation between the number of terminal branches and AVM size and a weak relationship with AVM location in the superficial or deep position. These two variables (size and location) are used in the subsequent analysis and the association between these variables and the number of terminal branches is a secondary argument when assessing the operability of an AVM.

Assessment of the risk for haemorrhage has been associated with, for example, AVM size. In most clinical series [12, 13, 15, 35, 41] small malformations have been associated with a relatively high incidence of haemorrhage. Some authors have therefore assumed that small AVM have a poorly adapted and fragile vascular bed on the venous side and that this explains their tendency to haemorrhage. When analysing clinical materials and discussing the properties of AVM which have bled, however, it is important to bear in mind that the material comprises only symptomatic AVM. It may be tempting to conclude that the risk of haemorrhage is greater with small AVM than with large AVM, but this conclusion cannot be drawn without knowledge of the actual number of asymptomatic AVM in a normal material. The prevalence of intracranial AVM in postmortem studies is higher than the prevalence of known, symptomatic AVM in the population [4]. The true number of patients with intracranial AVM is undoubtedly even higher, as postmortem examinations often do not include serial sections of the brain. It is possible that onset of other types than haemorrhage, e.g., epilepsy, only occurs in cases of AVM with a certain size and that a small AVM can only reveal its presence by haemorrhaging.

The analysis also shows that AVM giving clinical symptoms before the age of 30 years are usually situated in nonsilent areas, whereas symptomatic AVM after 30 years are usually situated in silent areas. Large AVM are more frequent in the latter age-group. This might suggest that AVM increases in size since growth can occur over longer periods in silent areas without giving symptoms. Only when it reaches a certain size will an AVM with this location give symptoms.

Our knowledge about which part of an AVM bleeds is uncertain. It does not seem likely that it is the arterial side but whether it is the abnormal vascular bundle or the often wide draining veins adjacent to it is unclear in most cases. What is more, it is often impossible to establish where the malformation ends and the venous side begins. It seems probable that the dilated veins gradually arterialize, i.e., develop thicker walls and adapt to the circulatory conditions. Dilatation of the arteries is undoubtedly an adaptive change owing to altered flow conditions, but whether dilatation of the veins is an adaptive change or is the result of elevated intravascular pressure is not clear. The backflow phenomenon, which has not previously been described, is of interest in this context as it might be a factor that should be considered when assessing the haemorrhage risk for an AVM. Our results suggest that AVM with backflow into diversionary veins are less likely to bleed than AVM lacking such backflow. We also have the impression that the backflow pheomenon is considerably commoner in AVM with a high shunt flow than in AVM with a low shunt flow. The reduced bleeding tendency in AVM with backflow might be due to a circulatory adaptation of the vascular bed, with a larger volume on the venous side, which in turn should mean a lower intravascular pressure.

III. The Original Clinical Decision

Luigi Pellettieri

Introduction

Opinions differ as to how AVM should be treated [23, 52]. Most neurosurgeons favour surgical treatment, although there is controversy concerning the criteria for selection of patients and surgical technique. Other neurosurgeons argue convincingly in favour of conservative treatment. It seems reasonable to advocate a treatment policy which allows selection of the most suitable therapy in each individual case. In most decision processes certain clinical variables are clearly more important than others. When evaluating a clinical decision it is therefore important to identify which clinical variables the decision is based on and to rank the variables in order of importance for the decision process.

The purpose of this study was to answer the following questions: Which variables were of importance for the decision process? How can we determine which variables were more important than others for this process? In order to obtain answers to these questions from all the information provided by our material, we have to analyse which variables governed the neurosurgeon's line of action and measure the importance of each variable for the decision process.

Patients and Methods

The study comprises 166 consecutive cases of intracranial AVM investigated and treated at the Department of Neurosurgery at Sahlgren Hospital in Gothenburg between 1953 and 1971. The patients have been described in Chapter II. The patients were divided into operable (patients subjected to surgery) and inoperable (patients not subjected to surgery) cases. The variables which formed the basis of the decision for or against operation have been taken from the case records. In cases in which the neurosurgeon decided not to operate, the reason is almost always stated or can be deduced indirectly. Factors favouring surgery are also sometimes stated.

Having identified the variables, we ranked them in order of importance for the decision process. This was done by analysing each variable in bipolar terms: the patients were divided into those below 40 years and those above 40 years of age, the AVM were divided into large and small malformations, as defined in Chapter II, etc. The "nonsilent area", however, according to the original decision

Table 2 a. *Ranking of Variables According to the Original Decision*

Variables		The original clinical decision						Difference in percent units
		Operated patients			Nonoperated patients			
		No. of cases	%	Difference in %	No. of cases	%	Difference in %	
AVM	small	101	80.1	+ 60.2	25	19.9		70.2
Size	large	18	45.0		22	55.0	+ 10	
AVM	superficial	74	77.8	+ 55.6	21	22.2		30.0
Location	deep	45	62.3	+ 25.6	26	36.7		
Age	< 40	76	77.5	+ 55.0	22	22.5		28.4
	> 40	43	63.3	+ 26.6	25	36.7		
Sex	female	53	79.1	+ 58.2	14	20.9		25.0
	male	66	66.6	+ 33.2	33	33.4		
Symptoms	SAH	71	77.1	+ 54.2	21	22.9		24.6
At onset	no SAH	48	64.8	+ 29.6	26	35.2		
Neurology	no deficit	68	75.5	+ 51.1	22	24.4		16.8
At admission	deficit	51	67.1	+ 34.3	25	32.8		
AVM	silent area	93	72.0	+ 44.0	36	28.0		3.4
Location	nonsilent area	26	70.3	+ 40.6	11	29.7		

includes only AVM situated in the motor region and fissura Sylvii. The percentage distribution of each pole for each variable between the "operable" and "inoperable" groups was then calculated. The percentage differences within the poles for each variable may be regarded as a numerical expression of the covariance of different variables with the decision.

The method may be illustrated with the following example: for the variable "AVM-size" (Table 2 a) 80.1% (101/126) of patients with small AVM underwent surgery, while 19.9% (25/126) did not. Of all the patients with large AVM, 45.0% (18/40) were operated upon, whereas 55.0% (22/40) were given conservative treatment. Expressed in percentage units, this means that the number of operated patients in the group with small AVM exceeds the number of non-operated patients by 60.2 percentage units. Conversely, in the large AVM group the number of patients given conservative treatment exceeds the number subjected to surgery by 10 percentage units. The interval between these two differences in percentage units (70.2%) constitutes a symbolic and relative measure of the importance of the AVM size in the original decision process, in that small AVM were generally considered more operable than large malformations.

The corresponding calculation for the variable "AVM location" gives 30,0 percentage units greater operability for patients with "superficial AVM" compared to patients with "deep AVM" (again according to the original decision). Comparison of these variables ("AVM-size" and "AVM location") shows that more importance (expressed in percentage units) has been attached to "AVM-size" than to "AVM location" when deciding which treatment approach to adopt (70,2% compared to 30,0%). Other variables have been compared and ranked in the same way.

Results

Identification of variables: 119 malformations were considered operable (71.6%) whereas 47 were judged to be inoperable (28.4%). The reason for not operating was stated directly or indirectly. Both AVM-variables and patient-variables have been considered but greater importance seems consistently to have been attached to the AVM variables. The frequency with which different variables are stated as the reason for the decision not to operate is given in Fig. 14. When surgery was carried out, the same variables may be assumed to have predominated. The following AVM variables were of importance for the decision: AVM-size, AVM location in deep or superficial zones and in silent or nonsilent areas. The following patient variables were of importance: patient's age, symptoms at onset and neurology at admission. In no case did the patient's sex seem to have affected the decision but this variable is still included as it has been found to be of importance in other medical contexts [36]. There are, of course, other variables, apart from those mentioned above, which may have been important in the individual case. In particular, the surgeon may have decided on a conservative approach in doubtful cases when the patient had a negative attitude to surgery without having definitely refused it.

When deciding for or against operation, the clinician has of course weighed these variables against one another. The importance of each individual variable for the decision process can also be traced, but it must be borne in mind that the variables influence one another. Among patients with small AVM, 80% were operated upon, whereas only 45% of patients with large AVM underwent surgery. 62% of AVM deeply located and 78% of superficially located AVM were extirpated. Location in silent or nonsilent areas had very little influence on the decision whether or not to operate. Thus, 72% of AVM in silent areas and 70% of AVM in nonsilent areas were

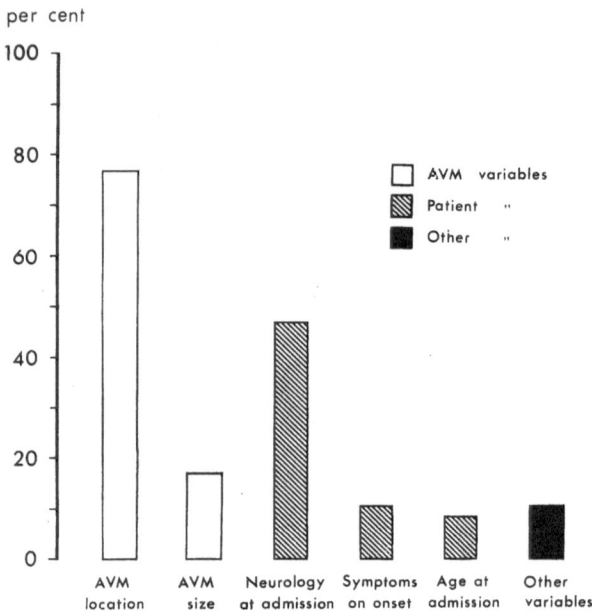

Fig. 14. Frequency with each variable was stated as the reason for not operating

extirpated. As regards the influence of neurology at admission, 76% of patients with normal neurology were operated upon, compared to 67% of the patients with deficits. Surgery was carried out in 77% of patients aged below 40 years, compared to 63% of those aged above 40. Women were subjected to surgery more often than men (79% compared to 66%). As regards the influence of the case history, 77% of patients with subarachnoidal haemorrhage (SAH) at onset were operated upon, compared to 65% of patients with other types of onset, e.g., epilepsy.

Ranking of variables: In the bipolar classification of the variables, the breakdown described in Chapter II has been used for AVM variables. Thus, AVM size has been divided into large (> 3 cm diameter) and small (< 3 cm diameter) and AVM location into superficial/deep and silent/nonsilent areas. As regards the patient variables, neurology at admission has been divided into no deficit (completely normal neurological findings) and deficit (some form of neurological disorder at admission). Patient age has been divided into below 40 and above 40 years. This age-limit was chosen because it seems to be decisive for the decision whether or not to operate as well as in the subsequent evaluation of the results (Chapters IV and V). When classifying the patients for the variable "symptoms at onset" the

Table 2 b. *Most Favourable and Most Unfavourable Risk Profile for Surgery According to the Original Clinical Decision*

Graded variables	Polarity favouring surgery	Polarity not favouring surgery
1—AVM-size	= small	large
2—AVM-location	= superficial	deep
3—Age at admission	= < 40	> 40
4—Sex	= female	male
5—Symptoms at onset	= SAH	no SAH
6—Neurology at admission	= no neurological deficit	neurological deficit
7—AVM-location	= silent area	nonsilent area

designations "SAH" and "no SAH" were used as haemorrhage at onset seems to represent the most important distinction. The SAH group includes both pure subarachnoidal haemorrhages and SAH with concomitant intracerebral haemorrhages. The "no SAH" group is very heterogeneous and comprises patients with epilepsy, headache, dizziness, tinnitus etc.

In Table 2 a, the variables have been ranked according to the method described above. The calculation shows that AVM size was the most important variable for assessment of operability. The other variables covaried with the decision in decreasing order of importance, as follows: AVM location in deep or superficial zones, the patient's age, sex, symptoms at onset, neurology at admission and location in silent/nonsilent areas. All variables together make up a "risk profile". In Table 2 b the two most extreme risk profiles for operability/inoperability, according to the original decision, are described. There are several other "risk profiles" between these two extremes. They represent patients who were judged to be operable to varying extent. Both favourable and unfavourable variables, in various combinations, are included in these risk profiles.

Discussion

According to the original decision, the ideal patient for operation is a woman, aged below 40 years, who had SAH at onset and almost normal neurology at admission. The AVM should be small and located superficially in a silent area. A mirror image of this pattern, made up of the opposite pole of each variable, gives the risk profile for patients who were considered least operable. Between these extremes there is a spectrum of other "risk profiles" which were judged to be more or less operable, depending on how the variables were combined. It is also clear that for each "risk profile" the variables influence one another, but this influence is difficult to measure.

The fact that patients aged below 40 years predominate among operated cases, for example, may be due either to their having been considered young enough for operation or to the fact that patients aged below 40 years more often had an SAH onset, which in turn means that they usually had small AVM (see Chapter IV). Both an SAH onset and the occurrence of small AVM were factors favouring operation.

The fact that women were more often operated upon than men might be explained by their younger age of onset than men or by their higher rate of SAH onset. Many factors may thus have interacted to make women seem more operable.

The finding that an SAH onset predominated among the operable cases may seem selfevident. It may, however, be due to the fact that SAH is more common at younger ages, in people with small AVM etc. On the other hand, the over-representation of epileptic onset among the inoperable patients may be due to their relatively high age and large AVM (see Chapter II). The finding that superficially located AVM were extirpated more often than deeply located malformations may also seem self-evident, but covariance with, for example, low age and small AVM may have influenced the decision here too.

In this study intracerebral hematomas (ICH) are not used as a separate variable. In most cases its presence is sufficiently manifested by means of other variables as "type of onset" and "neurology at admission". In a few cases an ICH has eliminated the importance of other variables in the decision process. This refers to patients who arrived in poor condition and/or presented deteriorating neurology and where acute surgery was considered necessary (see Chapter V). The treatment policy of ICH in connection with AVM is thus analogous to that proposed for spontaneous ICH and ICH ruptured arterial aneurysms.

The evaluation of the importance of different variables for the decision process reflects the clinician's experience. Only if this patient selection proves to give optimal results can the evaluation serve as a basis for criteria for management of AVM. The main aim of the following chapters of this work is to analyse the extent to which the original decision was correct or must be modified.

IV. Conservative Treatment

Luigi Pellettieri and Carl-Axel Carlsson *

Introduction

It is a generally accepted fact that patients with AVM are less likely to suffer fatal haemorrhage than patients with arterial aneurysms. Whatever one's views on the treatment of AVM, one has to accept that an AVM entails a potential risk to the patient's life or quality of life. If the AVM can be extirpated, this risk is eliminated. The question then arises whether the risk of operation is greater than the risk of conservative treatment. In order to answer this question it is necessary to study the natural history of patients with AVM.

In our series, as in other studies, the selection of patients for operation has been based on the clinician's assessment of the operability of the AVM (see Discussion, Chapter II). This means that it cannot be taken for granted that the malformations that would have been most likely to bleed were extirpated. This may have happened to be so, but the opposite situation may also apply. It might be assumed that if an operated group had been treated conservatively the risk for bleeding would be the same as in a group selected for conservative treatment. The results would then be directly comparable in the two groups of treatment. Selection for operation or conservative treatment applied here means, however, that the two groups are in fact so different that this line of reasoning is not tenable. The risk of haemorrhage may be assumed to depend on variables that are unequally distributed between the two groups—AVM-location, AVM-size, patient age etc. In order to be able to compare the operated and nonoperated group, identical patient-AVM constellations must therefore be used.

In this study the history of conservatively treated patients with AVM has been studied and the influence of different factors on the course has been analysed. The overall aim was to find out which patient-AVM constellations (risk profiles) were most favourable and

* Department of Neurosurgery, Sahlgren Hospital, University of Gothenburg, Gothenburg, Sweden.

which had an unfavourable influence on the prognosis. These different risk profiles will be compared in Chapter V with identical risk profiles in the group of operated patients.

As a background to the study, a brief review of previous reports on the natural history of patients with AVM will be given below. As the literature in this field is very extensive, only papers published during recent years will generally be discussed.

Previous Reports

As a rule, AVM manifests itself clinically by haemorrhaging or causing epilepsy, sometimes both. The haemorrhage may give rise to different symptoms, depending on its location and magnitude. Several other symptoms which are not directly attributable to this mechanism have been reported—dementia, headache, tinnitus etc.

Epilepsy was formerly considered to be the most common symptom of onset but in recent years haemorrhage as the first symptom has been increasingly often reported. Thus, Olivecrona and Riives [33] found SAH onset in only 40% of their patients, MacKenzie [24] in 30%, Paterson and McKissock [35] in 42%, and Tönnis et al. [53] in 33%. In later series, Perret and Nishioka [37] reported SAH-onset in 68% of their cases, Henderson and Gomez [12] in 76%, Troupp et al. [51] in 58%, Forster et al. [9] in 71%, and Nyström [31] in 55%.

This shift in favour of SAH-onset may be due to clinicians having become more observant of this diagnosis. Patients with SAH are increasingly often subjected to neuroradiological investigation nowadays, even when the onset is undramatic and the patient recovers relatively quickly after a headache and/or transient loss of consciousness, without subsequent neurological deficit. Many of these patients were formerly not subjected to radiological investigation. Patients with epileptic onset, on the other hand, have usually been subjected to extensive investigation.

The rate of epileptic onset has varied in different clinical series. Perret and Nishioka [37] found epileptic onset in 28% of their patients, Troupp et al. [51] in 24.8%, Forster et al. [9] in 47% and Nyström [31] in 17%.

A patient with a primary epileptic onset may suffer SAH later. According to Perret and Nishioka [37], this occurs in 18% of cases. The interval between epilepsy and SAH varies between 1 and 36 years. The opposite course, i.e., primary SAH-onset followed by epilepsy, occurs in 12.6% of patients, according to the same authors.

In addition to SAH and epilepsy, a number of other types of onset have been described in the literature. Perret and Nishioka [37] reported headache without verified SAH in 33 out of 55 cases.

Numbness, dysphasia, vertigo, ataxia, ptosis, mental confusion and tinnitus have also been reported as the first symptom. In a study of 137 patients with AVM, Troupp et al. [51] found migraine in 5 cases, headache and vertigo in 5 and "other symptoms" in one case. Nyström [31] reported headache in 17% of his series, tinnitus in 1% and "other symptoms" in 4%.

Perret and Nishioka [37] state the age of onset to be 10–20 years for SAH and 30–50 for epilepsy. Troupp et al. [51] found 31 years to be the peak age for onset of symptoms. Forster et al. [9] also state the peak age to be about 30 years for SAH-onset and 25 years for epileptic onset. Nyström [31] found that the onset occurred between the ages of 20 and 40 years in 52% of cases, irrespective of the type of onset. According to most authors, AVM is twice as common in men as in women [37].

AVM accounts for about 6% of all subarachnoidal haemorrhages [37]. The haemorrhage is generally not as massive as from an anterial aneurysm but may rather be described as effusion of blood [48]. According to Perret and Nishioka [37], 36% of SAH occur during sleep and 30.5% in connection with lifting, urination, defecation, coitus, cough or strong emotional experience. Trauma is stated to be the triggering factor in 4.4% and extracranial surgery in 0.5% of cases. Pregnancy is considered to increase the risk of haemorrhage in patients with AVM from the normal 10% to 87%. If an SAH caused by an AVM occurs during pregnancy, the risk of recurrence of haemorrhage during the same pregnancy is 27% [43].

Perret and Nishioka [37] reported 27 recurrences of haemorrhage in 103 nonoperated patients. The interval between the haemorrhages varied from a few days to several years. Forster et al. [9] stated that recurrence of haemorrhage occurs in 8–9% of nonoperated patients. Nyström [31] found that 15% of his nonoperated patients had one recurrence and 9% had had two or more recurrences of haemorrhage.

There seems to be some correlation between the type of onset and the location of the malformation. Tönnis et al. [53] state that patients presenting with epilepsy usually have an AVM located in the central or precentral gyrus. Perret and Nishioka [37] found that generalized seizures were more frequent in patients with lesions situated in the frontal area, while focal seizures predominated in those with lesions involving the parietal lobe.

There are several reports on the correlation between the type of onset and the size of the malformation. Hendersson and Gomez [12] found that all small AVM (2 cm or less in diameter) and 85.7% of those of medium size (2–6 cm) gave an SAH onset. Stehbens [48] claimed that the intensity of the haemorrhage and occurrence of intracerebral haematoma is greatest in individuals with small or medium-sized AVM. Similarly, Krayenbühl and Siebermann [16] reported SAH-onset in all of a group of 24 patients with small malformations. Nyström [8] has proposed a possible explanation why small AVM might bleed more often than large AVM. He points out that small malformations grow faster than large ones, which may lead to incompletely developed venous drainage from the small AVM. The intravascular pressure in these malformations would then be higher than in the large AVM. Paterson and McKissock [35] are of another opinion and consider that large malformations bleed just as often as small ones.

It is well known that SAH onset may give very different symptoms, apart from influencing consciousness. In a series of 247 patients with SAH-onset, Perret and Nishioka [37] found neurological deficits in 130 (53%): 90 patients had hemiparesis, 28 hemiplegia, 6 facial palsy, 2 dysphasia and 4 hemianopsia. In other materials neurological deficits have been found in 24% [12], 8.7% [51], 30% [9] and 18% [31]. Most of these cases of neurological deficit reported in the literature were accompanied by intracerebral haematoma. Intraventricular haemorrhage is a rare complication of AVM rupture. These haemorrhages generally occur from AVM protruding into the ventricular system [48]. Subdural haematoma is also a rare complication [28].

The mortality from SAH in nonoperated patients differs in different series: Svien and McRae [50] found a mortality rate of 6%, Perret and Nishioka [37] 10%, Troupp et al. [51] 10.2%, and Nyström [31] 20.4%. The long-term results in survivors are reported in the literature in terms of the neurological findings at controls and ability to work. Troupp et al. [51] refer to neurological findings and state that 55 of 116 surviving patients were well, 28 fairly well and 33 disabled. Perret and Nishioka [37] report that 23 out of 71 patients were well, 19 had minimal symptoms, 19 were partly handicapped but were able to work, 8 were unable to work but able to look after themselves and two were complete invalids. In Nyström's study [31] 34% of the patients had full working capacity, 28% partial working capacity and 17% no working capacity. Forster et al. [9] found that 60% of their patients had full working capacity, 31% reduced working capacity, 3% were unfit for regular employment but fully independent and mobile and 6% were chronic invalids.

Patients and Methods

The complete material described in Chapter II (166 patients) has been used in the analysis of the early case history, *i.e.*, type of onset and neurological findings at admission to hospital. For the late history, *i.e.*, late evolution and death, only the nonoperated patients have been studied (47 patients). The operated patients were thus studied together with the nonoperated group up to the point of operation. Information from case records includes the variables found to be important for the original decision for or against surgery in Chapter III: the patient's sex and age, the type of onset (SAH, epilepsy or "other onset"), the neurological finding at admission, the size and location of the AVM. The occurrence of intracerebral haematoma has been noted. Recurrences of haemorrhages and their time intervals have also been recorded. The mortality is presented as "short-term mortality" and "long-term mortality". "Short-term mortality" is defined as death immediately after onset and "long-term mortality" means death in connection with recurrence of haemorrhage.

In addition to the information obtained from case records, the patients have been followed up by letter and also by telephone. The average duration of follow-up was 10.5 years. The patient's neurological status has been classified as "no or slight neurological symptoms" or "moderate or severe neurological symptoms". Patients with slight neurological symptoms have been grouped with patients without any symptoms whatsoever as their symptoms were so slight or so diffuse that they could be regarded as relatively unimportant. These patients had, for example, headache, vertigo or well-controlled epilepsy. Each of the two groups was related to the seven variables, sex, age, type of onset, neurological findings at admission, AVM-locations and AVM-size. An attempt was also made to assess the long-term results in terms of ability to work, *i.e.*, whether the patient worked full-time or less than full-time.

Results

Mortality

Eight patients died, three immediately after onset of symptoms and five later from recurrence of haemorrhage. The short-termed mortality among nonoperated patients is thus 6.4% (3 out of 47). The percentage mortality from recurrence of haemorrhage (long-termed mortality) can only be calculated for the nonoperated patients who survived the first haemorrhage, *i.e.*, 40 patients (after allowing for three deaths from the first haemorrhage and four patients who could not be traced for follow-up). The long-term mortality is thus 12.5% (5 out of 40). These five patients died from recurrence of haemorrhage 5 years, 5 years, 9 years, 10 years, and 13 years after the first haemorrhage. Their data with respect to the variables under study are presented in Table 3 which also describes the three patients who died from their first haemorrhage. The postmortem examination showed that six of the eight patients who died had intracerebral haematomas, while two only had subarachnoidal haemorrhage with cerebral swelling.

Table 3. *Relationships Between the Causes of Death and Other Variables*

Cause of death	Age	Sex	Symptoms at onset	Neurological findings (deficit or no deficit)	AVM-size (large or small)	AVM-location (superficial or deep)	AVM-location (silent or nonsilent area)
ICH (first bleeding)	18	female	SAH	deficit	small	deep	silent
SAH (first bleeding)	14	male	SAH	deficit	large	deep	silent
SAH (first bleeding)	57	male	Jackson-epilepsy other	deficit	small	superficial	nonsilent
ICH (rebleeding)	16	male	symptoms	deficit	large	deep	silent
ICH (rebleeding)	35	male	SAH	deficit	small	deep	silent
ICH (rebleeding)	45	female	SAH	deficit	large	deep	nonsilent
ICH (rebleeding)	45	male	SAH	deficit	small	superficial	silent
ICH (rebleeding)	69	male	Jackson-epilepsy	deficit	large	deep	nonsilent

Type of Onset

The percentage distribution by type of onset is given in Fig. 15. SAH-onset dominates (55%), followed by epileptic onset (34%) and "other types of onset" (11%). "Other types of onset" include mental disorders, headache, blurred vision, vertigo etc. The SAH-group includes 28 patients with intracerebral haematoma (ICH) (30%). The distribution by type of epilepsy in the epileptic onset group is as follows: 72% grand mal, 22% Jacksonian epilepsy and 6% grand mal combined with Jacksonian epilepsy. In four cases the onset of grand mal was simultaneous with SAH. Simultaneous onset of Jacksonian epilepsy and SAH did not occur.

Five patients with epileptic onset subsequently suffered SAH. The time interval between epileptic onset and SAH varied between 1 and 33 years. In seven patients the course was the opposite, *i.e.*, SAH-onset was later followed by epilepsy. The time interval for this course varied between 1 and 32 years. In our series of 92 SAH, 23 patients (25%) suffered 30 recurrences of haemorrhage. The time relationship between the primary haemorrhage and recurrrences is shown in Fig. 16. Recurrence of haemorrhage occurred on an average 7.3 years after primary haemorrhage but there was a wide variation, with a range from 9 weeks to 30 years. For the patients with epileptic onset, the time interval between the first epileptic seizure and recurrence of seizure was on average 10.3 years. Epileptic seizures were found to occur in periods, with a tendency towards regular attack-free intervals.

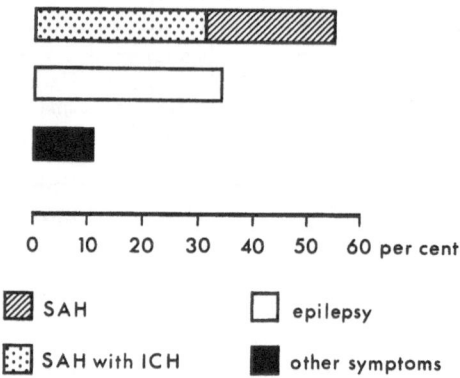

Fig. 15. Percentages of various diagnoses at admission

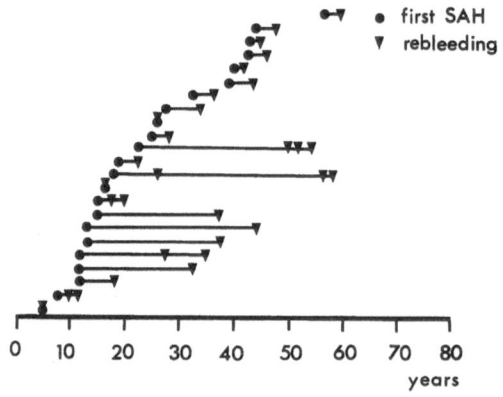

Fig. 16. Time elapsing between first SAH and rebleeding, versus age, in 23 nonoperated patients

Intracerebral haematoma occurred in 28 patients (30.4% of the 92 patients with SAH-onset). The distribution of intracerebral haematoma *versus* age showed a peak between 20 and 40 years. No great difference in sex distribution could be found. In four patients intracerebral haematoma was diagnosed at admission, while in 16 patients the symptoms were interpreted as subarachnoidal haemor-

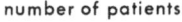

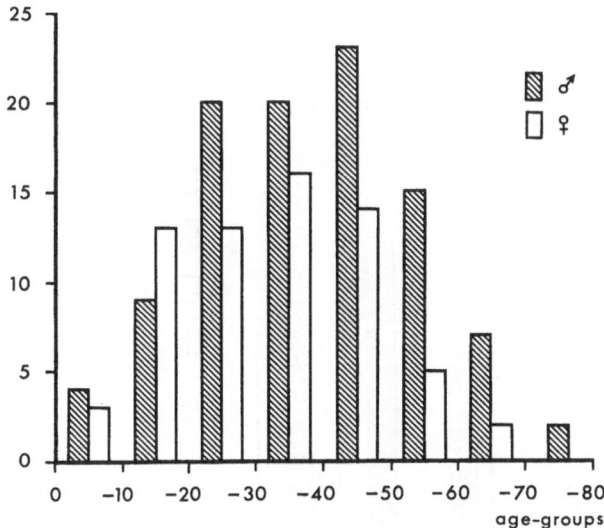

Fig. 17. Distribution of male and female patients, versus age

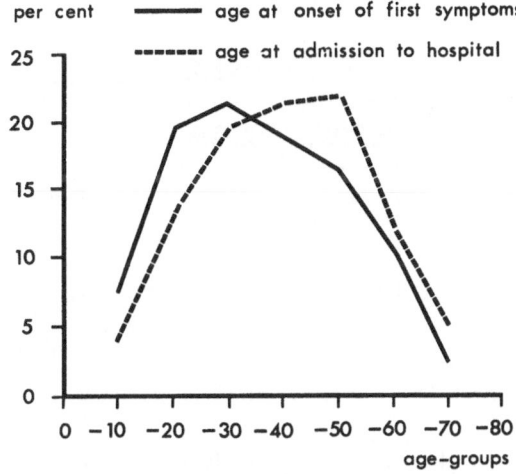

Fig. 18. Distribution of AVM-patients versus age at onset of first symptoms and age at admission to hospital

rhage without an expansive lesion. Two patients only had epileptic seizures (grand mal), without clinical signs of subarachnoidal haemorrhage. Six patients died and the diagnosis was established at the postmortem examination.

Relationships Between the Variables

Type of onset versus age and sex: The age and sex distribution at admission of the patients is shown in Fig. 17. Men predominate (60%). Fig. 18 shows the distribution by age at onset and age at admission. Age at onset shows a peak between 20 and 30 years. The

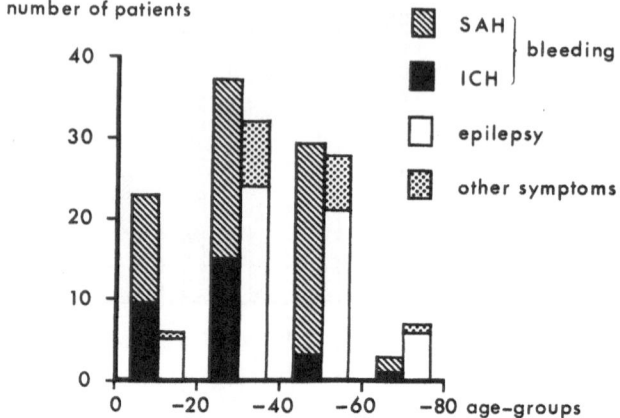

Fig. 19. Distribution of various diagnoses at admission, versus age

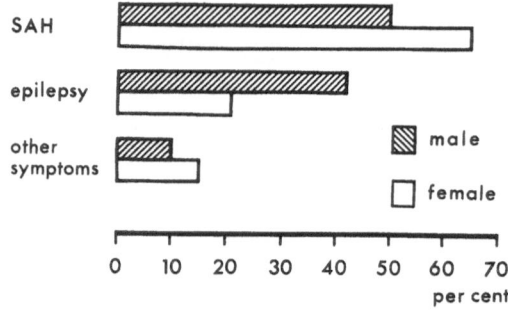

Fig. 20. Distribution of various diagnoses, versus sex

distance between the two curves reflects the average time interval between the first symptoms and admission to hospital. Fig. 19 shows the distribution by age at admission for the two main types of onset—haemorrhage and no haemorrhage. It will be seen that SAH-onset is more common than epileptic onset in age-groups up to 20 years. At higher ages there is a tendency towards equalization of the distribution but SAH continues to dominate up to the fifth decade. Fig. 20 shows the percentage distribution by type of onset

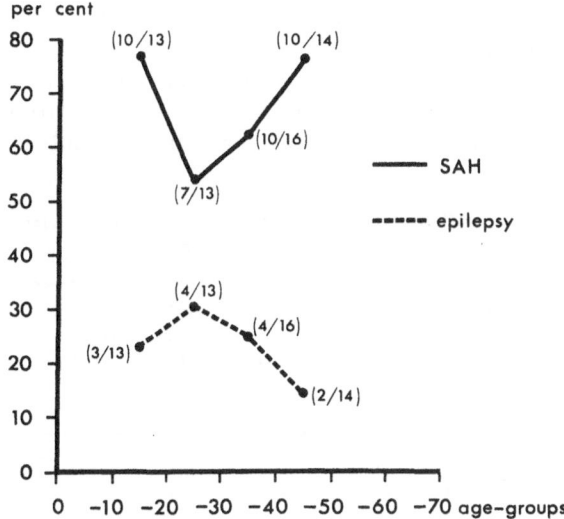

Fig. 21. Symptoms at onset (SAH and epilepsy), versus age, in female patients

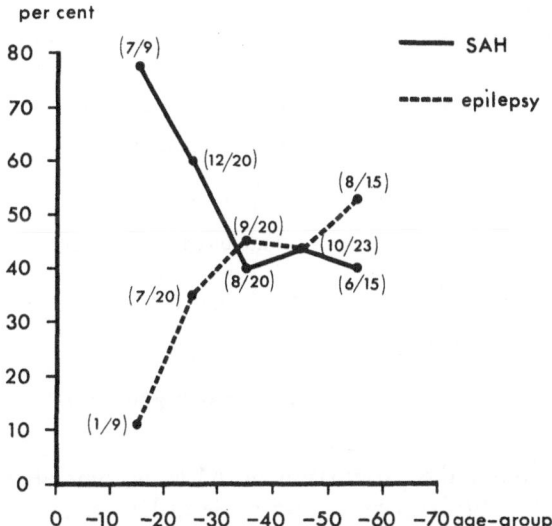

Fig. 22. Symptoms at onset (SAH and epilepsy), versus age, in male patients

versus sex. Women are more frequent among patients with SAH while men more often have epileptic onset. Figs. 21 and 22 show the distribution by SAH and epileptic onset in women and men *versus* age. It will be seen that women account for most cases of SAH onset up to 30 years of age and men account for most cases of epileptic onset after 30 years of age.

Type of onset versus AVM-locations and AVM-size: In patients with SAH-onset the proportion of AVM in the frontal lobe and occipital lobe is somewhat greater than in other lobes. In patients

Table 4. *Relationships Between AVM-Locations in Different Areas of the Brain and Symptoms at Onset*

Symptoms at onset	Frontal lobe	Motor area and fissura Sylvii	Tem- poral lobe	Parietal lobe	Temporo- parieto- occipital area	Occi- pital lobe	Poste- rior fossa	Skull base	Intra- ven- tricular	Total number of patients
SAH	22	18	9	10	5	15	4	6	3	92
Epilepsy	16	16	6	11	2	5	0	0	0	56
Other symptoms	4	3	2	2	0	6	0	1	0	18
Total number of patients	42	37	17	23	7	26	4	7	3	166

Table 5. *Relationships Between AVM-Sizes and Bleeding at Onset*

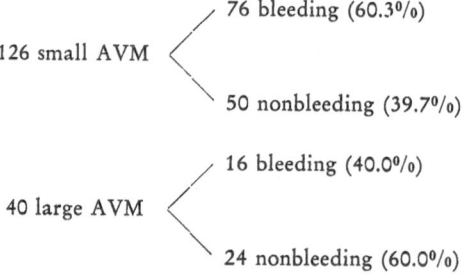

126 small AVM
 76 bleeding (60.3%)
 50 nonbleeding (39.7%)

40 large AVM
 16 bleeding (40.0%)
 24 nonbleeding (60.0%)

with epileptic onset the proportion of AVM is somewhat greater in the frontal lobe, Sylvian fissure and parietal lobe than in other lobes (Table 4). Superficially located malformations are somewhat more frequent than deeply located (57 and 43% respectively). Deeply located AVM seem to have a somewhat greater tendency to bleed than those located superficially (60 and 51% respectively) (Fig. 23). For patients with epileptic onset, there is no marked difference between deeply and superficially located AVM (32 and 35% respectively).

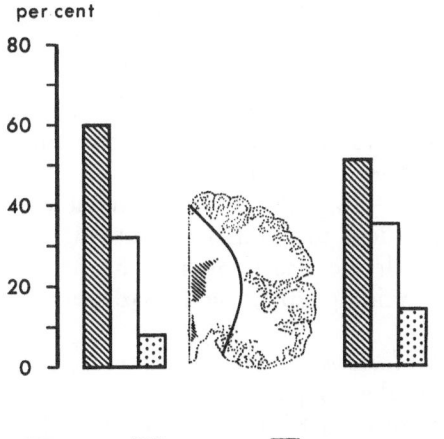

per cent

Fig. 23. Distribution of various diagnoses according to AVM-location
(deep and superficial)

Table 6. *Relationships Between Symptoms at Onset and Neurological Findings
at Admission*

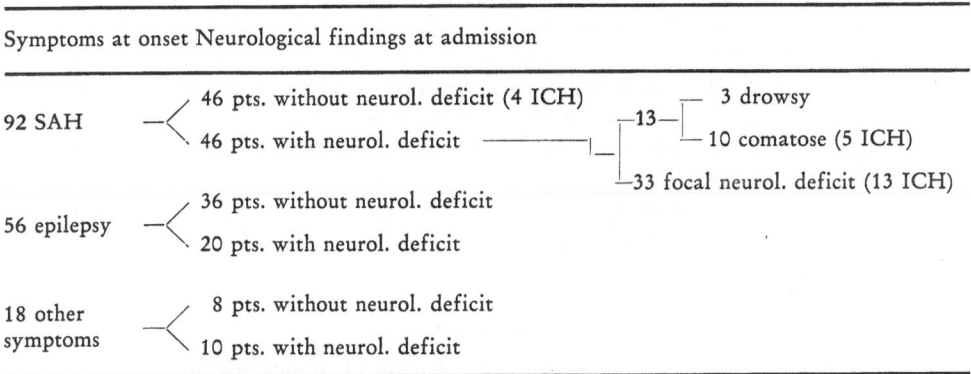

Symptoms at onset Neurological findings at admission

92 SAH	46 pts. without neurol. deficit (4 ICH)	3 drowsy
	46 pts. with neurol. deficit — —13—	10 comatose (5 ICH)
		33 focal neurol. deficit (13 ICH)
56 epilepsy	36 pts. without neurol. deficit	
	20 pts. with neurol. deficit	
18 other symptoms	8 pts. without neurol. deficit	
	10 pts. with neurol. deficit	

The relationship between type of onset and AVM-size is shown
in Table 5. 126 AVM were classed as small (Chapter II). Seventysix
of these malformations (60%) bled, whereas 50 (40%) did not lead
to SAH-onset. Forty of the malformations were classed as large.
Sixteen (40%) of them caused SAH-onset and 24 (60%) did not.
Twentyfive of the large malformations were very large (more than
4 cm in diameter). Six of these very large AVM caused SAH-onset
and 19 did not.

Type of onset versus neurological findings at admission: Ninety patients (54%) did not exhibit neurological deficits at onset, while 76 patients (46%) were found to have neurological deficits. The group with neurological deficits includes patients with reduced level of consciousness only. Ninetytwo patients (55%) had SAH-onset. Fortysix of them had no neurological deficit at admission despite the fact that four patients had ICH. Of the SAH-patients with neurological deficits (46), three were somnolent and ten were comatose. Five of these ten comatose patients had ICH. Of the 56 patients with epileptic onset, 36 had no neurological deficit at admission. The remaining 20 patients had persistent symptoms of deficit type (Table 6).

Neurological findings at admission versus age, sex, AVM-location and AVM-size: Of the 90 patients without neurological deficits at admission, 58% were aged below 40 years and 42% were 40 years or older. Of the 76 patients with neurological deficits at admission, 61% were aged below 40 years and 39% were aged 40 years or above.

39% of female patients were found to have neurological deficits, compared with 49% of the males.

Neurological deficits were commonest in patients with AVM located in the motor region: 23 out of 37 patients with this AVM-location had neurological deficits. Of the 90 patients without neurological deficits at admission, 60% had superficially located AVM. The AVM was superficially located in 54% of the 76 patients who had neurological deficits at admission. There was a certain relation between neurological findings at admission and AVM-size: 80% of the 90 patients without neurological deficits at admission had small AVM while 20% had large AVM. Of the 76 patients with neurological deficits at admission, 71% had small AVM and 29% had large AVM.

Outcome

For obvious reasons, only the 47 (28%) nonoperated patients could be included in the study of the subsequent course of the disease and long-term results. Four patients could not be traced and the analysis of the long-term results is therefore based on 43 patients. Three of these 43 patients died from the first haemorrhage and five from recurrence of haemorrhage (see above). Analysis of the distribution by neurological findings for the 35 surviving patients showed that 15 patients had no or slight neurological symptoms (43%) and 20 patients had moderate or severe neurological symptoms (57%) (Table 7).

All patients in the group with no or slight neurological symptoms were working full-time. In the group with moderate or severe neurological symptoms, 60% were working full-time: the remaining patients were working only part-time or were not working at all (Table 7).

Table 7. *Relationships Between Neurological Findings at Admission and Long-Term Results in Nonoperated Patients*

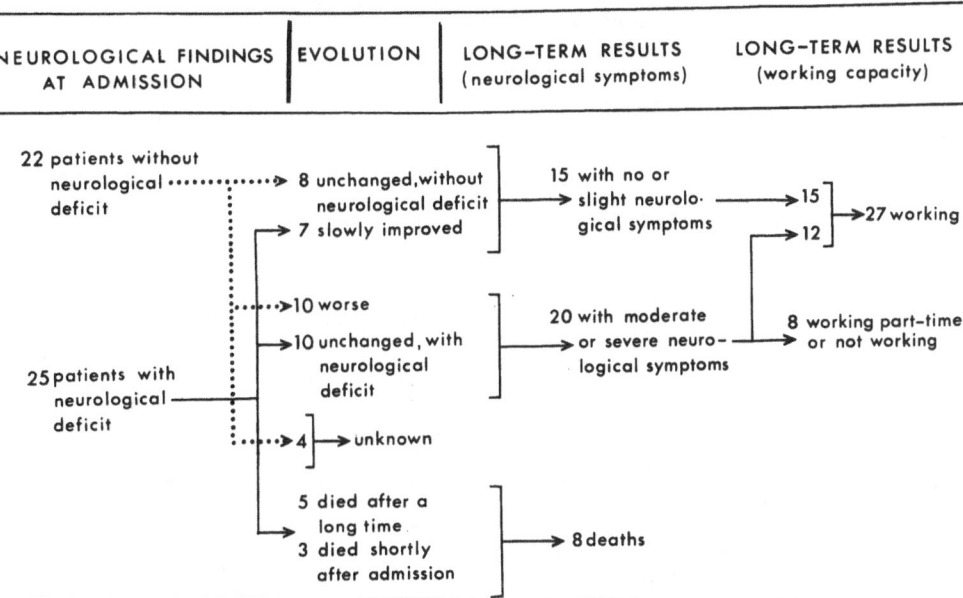

Ranking of Variables

The different variables studied influence the prognosis to differing extent. As in Chapter III, each variable was described in bipolar terms, *i.e.*, the patient's age was classified as above 40 or below 40 years, AVM-size as large or small etc. etc. The percentage distribution of the two poles of each variable in the groups "no or slight neurological symptoms" and "moderate or severe neurological symptoms" was calculated. The differences in percentage units within each bipole may be considered to represent a numerical measure of the covariance of each variable with the results. The variable which exhibits the greatest difference in percentage units between its poles was thus considered to have the greatest prognostic value. The variable with the next greatest difference was ranked number 2, and so on. The ranking of the variables is illustrated in Table 8 a.

Table 8 a. *Relationships Between Percentages of Good and Poor Results and Different Variables (Placed in Order of Per Cent Differences). Long-Term Follow-Up of 43 Nonoperated Patients (Each Variable is Divided in Two Poles)*

Variables		Long-term results						
		No or slight neurological symptoms		Moderate or severe neurological symptoms			Value of signifi-cance	Level of signifi-cance	Difference in percent-age units
		No. of cases	%	No. of cases	%	differ-ence in %			
Age at admission	< 40	11	50.0	11	50.0	± 0	0	0	
	> 40	4	20.0	17	80.0	+ 60.0	3.44	***	60.0
Neurology at admission	no deficit	9	50.0	9	50.0	± 0	0	0	
	deficit	6	24.0	19	76.0	+ 52.0	2.92	**	52.0
AVM-location	superficial	8	47.0	9	53.0	+ 6.0	0	0	
	deep	7	27.0	19	73.0	+ 46.0	2.70	**	40.0
AVM-location	silent area	13	39.4	20	60.6	+ 21.2	0	0	
	non-silent area	2	20.0	8	80.0	+ 60.0	2.37	*	38.8
AVM-size	large	7	31.8	15	68.2	+ 36.4	0	0	
	small	8	38.0	13	62.0	+ 24.0	0	0	12.4
Sex	female	5	38.4	8	61.6	+ 23.2	0	0	
	male	10	33.3	20	66.6	+ 33.3	1.98	*	10.1
Symptoms at onset	no SAH	8	34.7	15	65.0	+ 30.0	0	0	
	SAH	7	35.0	13	65.3	+ 30.6	0	0	0.6

  * 0.01 < p < 0.05.
  ** 0.001 < p < 0.01.
  *** p < 0.001.

Age proved to be the most important factor for the prognosis, followed by the neurological findings at admission, AVM-location (superficial or deep) etc. The results were thus consistently better in patients aged below 40 years, patients without neurological deficits at admission, patients with superficially located malformations, patients with malformations in silent areas, and so on. In patients with moderate or severe neurological symptoms the above variables showed the opposite polarity, *i.e.,* these patients were usually above 40 years of age, had neurological deficits at admission and had malformations located deeply, and so on (Table 8 b). Between these extremes there were a number of intermediate risk profiles which had a more or less favourable pattern of combination of variables. It is also clear that the variables within each risk profile influence one another in a way that is difficult to measure.

Table 8 b. *Most Favourable and Most Unfavourable Risk Profile For Good Results (Nonoperated Patients)*

Graded variables	Polarity favourable for good results	Polarity unfavourable for good results
Age at admission	= < 40	> 40
Neurology at admission	= no neurological deficit	— neurological deficit
AVM-location	= superficial	— deep
AVM-location	= silent area	— nonsilent area
AVM-size	= small	— large
Sex	= female	— male
Symptoms at onset	= SAH	— no SAH

Discussion

The study has shown that different patient-AVM constellations (risk profiles) are differently distributed with respect to the long-term results in nonoperated patients. This was the main purpose of the analysis as these profiles will be matched with identical profiles in the operated group in Chapter V. Patients with identical profiles in the two groups can thus be compared since the effect of the original selection for operation or conservative treatment is thereby reduced. This procedure obviates the sources of error which seem to influence previous investigations, in which the results in the whole groups of operated and nonoperated patients have been compared directly. It would naturally be interesting to know how great the error is in such a direct comparison. We have endeavoured to estimate this error from the results of our study by applying the following line of reasoning: the selection of patients is based on judgement of the operability of the malformation. In addition, SAH was considered to be a stronger indication for surgery than other types of onset. Both these factors may, but need not necessarily, mean a difference in outcome between the groups. In other words, would the patients who were submitted to surgery have had a different prognosis from those selected for conservative treatment if they had not been operated upon? A tentative answer to this question can be obtained by an indirect test. It is incontestable that all 166 patients in the original series "received" conservative treatment up until admission. The average history in these patients was about 10 years. Their condition at admission may therefore be considered to represent the long-term results in an unselected group of patients with AVM who were "treated" conservatively. If the morbidity in this group of 166 "unselected" patients is compared with that in the group of 47 patients selected for conservative treatment, the distribution by morbidity in the two groups is practically identical (66% morbidity in the 166 "unselected" patients; 65% morbidity in the 47 patients selected for conservative treatment). This equal morbidity suggests that the natural course of the disease was not markedly changed by the selection as such. It may therefore be concluded that the investigators who have made direct comparisons between operated and nonoperated groups have consciously or unconsciously compared two fairly similar groups. Nonetheless, the possibility that the selection influences the results cannot be ruled out, as the nonoperated group at the time of selection contains fewer high-risk patients (*i.e.*, patients with SAH-onset) than the operated group.

Moreover it must be remembered that an unknown number of patients died outside the group studied and that the patients studied, up until admission to hospital, are the survivors from a larger group of unknown size. Our approach of comparing patients with identical profiles in the two groups therefore seems more reliable.

The mortality due to recurrence of heamorrhage in our patients is 12.5%. Perret and Nishioka [37] found the mortality from recurrence of haemorrhage in patients given conservative treatment to be 12%. The average survival after the first haemorrhage in patients who later died from recurrence of haemorrhage in our study is 5.5 years.

The female dominance in the group with SAH-onset is an interesting finding. SAH-onset in women occurs most often in the age-group 10–30 years. No woman aged above 50 presented with SAH in our series. It might be speculated that hormonal factors are of importance in this context since SAH-onset occurs in women of child-bearing age. It is known that cardiac output is increased during pregnancy, with a consequent increased load on AVM and increased risk of haemorrhage [43]. Perret and Nishioka [37] also found that women with AVM presenting with haemorrhage were younger than men. Note that up to 20 years of age the number of men and women in the material is practically equal. The greater number of SAH in this age-group is therefore attributed to the age factor and not due to over-representation of women. In our series, patients below 20 years of age usually had an SAH-onset, while above the age of 20 the disease usually presented with epilepsy or other types of onset. This may be explained by the fact that small AVM are more common in younger age-groups and that these small AVM are more likely to bleed than large AVM. Large AVM seem to have a greater tendency to cause epilepsy. Patients presenting with SAH may subsequently develop epilepsy. These patients do not generally suffer recurrence of haemorrhage. On the other hand, there are a few patients who primarily present with epilepsy but subsequently suffer SAH. This means that an epileptic primary onset is no guarantee that SAH will not occur later. Our study suggests, however, that if an AVM has not bled before the age of 20 years a nonhaemorrhage onset is more likely than SAH-onset, and that the risk for SAH-onset declines with age.

Of the patients with SAH-onset in our series, 25% suffered recurrence of haemorrhage. This recurrence rate is slightly higher than that reported by Perrèt and Nishioka [37] (23%). The average interval between primary SAH and recurrence in our patients was 7.3 years. Bleeding from an AVM is generally less massive than from arterial aneurysms. This difference is reflected in the clinical findings: intracerebral haemtatoma was diagnosed in only 14.3% of cases at admission. In the other cases, subarachnoidal haemorrhage without an expansive lesion was suspected. The reason is that the haematoma did not markedly influence the level of consciousness and that neurological deficits were generally slight or absent. Neurological deficits occurring without underlying intracerebral haematoma may have been due to vasospasm. The spasm could be demonstrated at angiography in only two patients. Spasm may, however, have been overlooked in several patients as this phenomenon is difficult to assess in patients with AVM, owing to the varying calibre of the feeding vessels.

Deeply located AVM have a somewhat greater tendency to bleed than those located superficially. The explanation for this is not clear. It is possible that it is due to the fact that AVM close to the midline are supplied by a larger number of arteries and have poorer drainage. This would mean an increased intravascular pressure in these AVM.

The degree of restitution was assessed in terms of ability to work and neurological findings. It was found that 77% of the patients were able to work full-time. 44% of these patients had moderate or severe neurological symptoms. We were therefore obliged to distinguish between the long-term results in terms of neurological findings and the ability of the patient to work. In our opinion, the neurological findings are the most appropriate measure of the condition of the patient. The fact that a patient with hemiplegia or severe epilepsy, after expensive and prolonged rehabilitation, can resume working is due to the special community in which the patient lives and the resources it provides. If the results are analysed in relation to ability to work, nonoperated AVM is a relatively benign disease from a social point of view (77% of the patients were working full-time). If, on the other hand, the results are assessed in terms of late neurological findings, conservatively treated AVM is a serious disease with a rather high morbidity (57% of the patients had neurological deficits).

The assessment was thus based exclusively on the neurological findings. 43% of the patients had no or slight neurological symptoms and 57% had moderate or severe neurological symptoms. By relating these results to the seven variables (age, sex, AVM-size, AVM-locations, symptoms at onset, and neurological findings at admission) it was possible to grade the variables with respect to prognostic importance. This grading was used to construct a risk profile for each patient.

The most favourable risk profiles for the prognosis in these conservatively treated patients show certain similarities to the profiles shown in Chapter III to be most likely to lead to the surgeon's deciding to operate. There are also certain similarities between these risk profiles and those which gave the best surgical results (Chapter V). This similarity between risk profiles which are favourable for the prognosis, irrespective of whether or not the patient is operated upon, has led to misunderstanding in the debate on treatment of AVM. A possible explanation for this situation will be discussed in the next chapter.

V. Surgical Treatment

Luigi Pellettieri, Carl-Axel Carlsson, and Gösta Norlén *

Introduction

The aim of this study was to identify which patient-AVM constellations (risk profiles) were favourable and which were unfavourable for the outcome after surgical treatment of AVM. These risk profiles will be matched against identical risk profiles in patients given conservative treatment. This reduces the effect of the original selection and makes it possible to compare the two forms of treatment.

As background to the study, some earlier, representative studies of surgical treatment of AVM will be reviewed. Although these studies are informative, comparison between different isolated series on the basis of the results alone are misleading as the results of surgical treatment are highly dependent on the criteria applied for selection. This applies to both comparisons between different operated series and comparisons between surgically and conservatively treated patients. Theoretically, it is of course possible to reduce the mortality and morbidity in an operated group to zero if only the most favourable cases are selected for operation. It may be assumed, however, that the surgeons in the series concerned endeavoured to operate all patients they considered operable but included an assessment of the risk for haemorrhage in their judgement. This latter variable means that the group of operated patients probably includes more high-risk patients than the nonoperated group. Consequently, the surgically and conservatively treated groups differ in composition. Direct comparison between the two groups is therefore misleading, although the error may be comparatively small (see Discussion Chapter IV).

Previous Reports

There are several different approaches to the treatment of AVM. They may be divided into extra- and intracranial procedures. The

* Professor in Neurosurgery, Head of the Department of Neurosurgery, Sahlgren Hospital, University of Gothenburg, Gothenburg, Sweden, 1953—1973. Present address: Linnégatan 35, Stockholm, Sweden.

extracranial procedures include irradiation of malformations, ligature of the carotid artery in the neck, with or without postoperative irradiation, and artificial embolization. The intracranial procedures include stereotactic surgery, cryosurgery, ligature of feeding arteries and total extirpation of the malformation.

Over the years several reports on treatment of series of patients with AVM by surgical extirpation have been published. Olivecrona and Riives [33] described a series of 60 patients, 24 of whom were treated by total extirpation. The operative mortality was 13% and one third of the operated patients became "practically well, with full earning capacity", one third had "defects but were practically able to work", and the remaining were "severely handicapped". Norlén [28] described 10 cases treated by total extirpation of the AVM. His operative mortality was zero and nine of the patients were in good condition and able to work full-time at follow-up, whereas only one patient had neurological deficits and was unable to work.

After these pioneer studies, larger series were described. Paterson and McKissock [35] described a series of 110 operated patients, 36 of whom underwent total extirpation. Four of these patients died, three were incapacitated and nine had slight deficits, while the remaining patients were well and able to work full-time. Eleven patients were treated by irradiation only. One-third of them died owing to haemorrhage and about half of the remainder were incapacitated with the passage of years. Olivecrona and Landenheim [32] described a series of 125 angiomas, 81 of which were totally excised. Seven of these patients died, 50 became completely well, 15 were improved and 7 deteriorated. Tönnis [54] described a series of 134 AVM, 56 of which were totally extirpated. Five patients died. 61% of the survivors had full working capacity, 22% were partially employed and 11% were invalids. The results in these early series are rather consistent, with an operative mortality between 5 and 10% and clinical improvement in about 85%.

Similar results have been reported in more modern series, in which refined surgical techniques have evidently compensated for broadening of the indications for surgery. Perret and Nishioka [37] described 148 surgical cases, 119 of which were treated by total resection. Thirteen of these patients died and 106 survived the operation. Eighty-five of these 106 patients were available for follow-up. Twenty-five of them became symptomless, 28 had minimal symptoms, 16 were partly incapacitated but capable of working, 11 were incapable of working but capable of looking after themselves and five patients were complete invalids. Forster et al. [9] report results from 95 operated cases. 60% of the patients became completely well,

21% had slight neurological deficits, with reduced working capacity, 11% had major neurological deficits but were able to look after themselves and 4% had serious neurological deficits and were totally incapable of looking after themselves. The operative mortality was 4%. Nyström [31] described 88 operated patients: 43% could be restored to "full working capacity", 23% to "partial working capacity" and 23% had "no working capacity". Eleven per cent of the patients died, 6% of them owing to recurrence of haemorrhage.

Patients and Methods

The study comprises 119 consecutive patients operated upon for AVM (see Chapter II). All the patients were treated at the Department of Neurosurgery, Sahlgren Hospital, Gothenburg during the 18-year period 1953–1971. The data were obtained from the case records and correspond to the data included in the study of non-operated patients (see Chapter IV). The collection of information also includes postoperative complications, such as postoperative haematoma, and reoperation. Postoperative angiographic control was performed in all patients. Most of the patients underwent total extirpation of the AVM. The surgical technique is the same as that described by Olivecrona and Riives [33]. The prognostic importance of different variables was calculated by the same method as was used for the nonoperated group (Chapter IV).

Results

Operative Findings

112 patients underwent total extirpation of the malformation (94%) and seven partial extirpation (6%). Intracerebral haematomas in connection with the malformation were found in 22 patients (18%). None of the operated patients had intraventricular haematomas. Subdural haematomas were found in two cases. Five arterial aneurysms were diagnosed at preoperative angiography, corresponding to 3% of the total series of 166 cases of AVM. In two of these cases the haemorrhage was interpreted as being caused by the arterial aneurysm and the aneurysm was ligatured in connection with extirpation of the AVM in both cases. Twelve patients were reoperated owing to postoperative haematoma. No other immediate postoperative complications which can be strictly ascribed to the operation were observed.

Mortality

The mortality is shown in Table 9. Sixteen out of 119 operated patients died (13%).

Nine patients died immediately after the operation. Three of these patients had ICH and were comatose at admission. They died

Table 9. *Relationships Between the Causes of Death and Other Variables*

Cause of death	Age	Sex	Symptoms at onset	Neurological findings (deficit or no deficit)	AVM-size (large or small)	AVM-location superficial or deep	AVM-location (silent or nonsilent area)
ICH at admission	30	male	SAH	deficit	small	superficial	nonsilent
ICH at admission	55	male	SAH	deficit	small	deep	nonsilent
ICH at admission	63	male	SAH	deficit	small	deep	silent
Huge operative bleeding	2	male	Grand mal	deficit	small	superficial	nonsilent
Huge operative bleeding	50	female	SAH	deficit	small	superficial	silent
Huge operative bleeding	56	male	Jackson-epi.	deficit	small	superficial	nonsilent
Postoperative haematoma	22	male	SAH	deficit	small	deep	nonsilent
Postoperative haematoma	34	male	Jackson-epi.	deficit	large	deep	nonsilent
Postoperative haematoma	34	female	Grand mal	deficit	large	superficial	silent
Bleeding from art. aneurysm	17	male	SAH	no deficit	small	deep	nonsilent
Rebleeding	37	male	SAH	no deficit	small	deep	nonsilent
Rebleeding	60	male	SAH	no deficit	small	deep	silent
Other causes	27	male	SAH	no deficit	small	deep	nonsilent
Other causes	48	male	Grand mal	no deficit	small	superficial	nonsilent
Other causes	45	male	Grand mal	deficit	small	superficial	silent
Other causes	47	male	SAH	no deficit	small	deep	silent

a few hours after the operation. Three patients died from uncontrollable haemorrhage during operation. The remaining three patients died during the first few days after the operation owing to postoperative haematoma in the operation wound. Seven patients died a long time after the operation. The cause of death is known for five of them: two patients died 2 and 2.5 years after the operation owing to recurrent haemorrhage from partially extirpated AVM;

one patient with a radically extirpated AVM died 2 years post-operatively owing to haemorrhage from a previously undetected arterial aneurysm. Two patients died from malignant disease. The causes of death in the remaining two cases were recorded as insufficiencia cordis and cerebrovascular insult, but no postmortem examination was performed. The cause of death, age, sex, type of onset, neurology at admission to hospital and AVM-size and AVM-locations for the patients who died are given in Table 9.

Relationships Between the Variables

Type of onset versus age and sex: The SAH-group is largest (60%), followed by the epileptic group (30%) and the group with other types of onset (10%) (Fig. 24). The latter group includes pa-

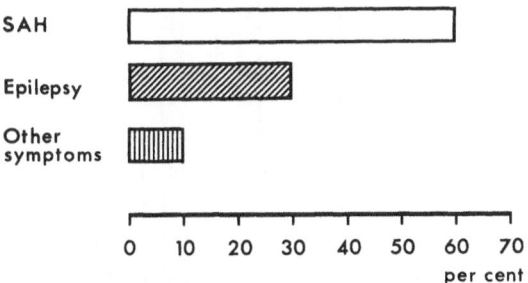

Fig. 24. Distribution of various diagnoses at admission

tients who presented with mental disturbances, headache, blurred vision, vertigo etc.

The distribution by age and sex is shown in Fig. 25. In the younger age-groups (below 20 years) women predominate, while men are somewhat over-represented in the age-groups above 20 years. A higher proportion of the women (79%) than of the men (67%) were subjected to surgery.

The relationship between SAH-onset and epileptic and other types of onset on the one hand and age on the other is shown in Fig. 26. Up to the fourth decade, SAH-onset was more common than non-SAH onset.

Analysis of the relationship between type of onset and sex shows that 37 men and 34 women presented with SAH. Among the patients with epileptic onset there is a marked male dominance (24 men compared to 12 women). Six men and six women had other types of onset.

Type of onset versus AVM-locations and AVM-size: The AVM-location and type of onset in the 119 operated patients with AVM is shown in Table 10. In the 71 patients who presented with SAH, the AVM was superficially located in 42 and deeply located in 29. Of the 36 patients with epileptic onset, 24 had superficially located

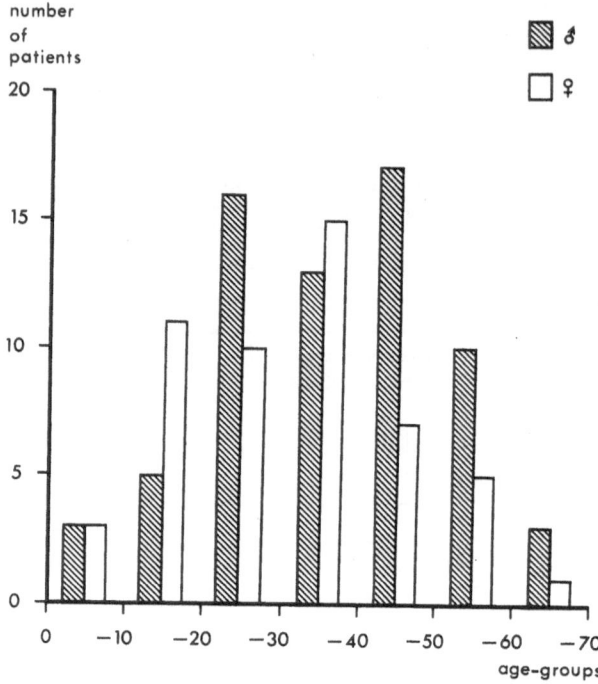

Fig. 25. Distribution of male and female patients, versus age

Table 10. *Relationships Between AVM-Locations in Different Areas of the Brain and Symptoms at Onset*

Location	Symptoms at onset			Total
	SAH (incl. ICH)	Epilepsy	Other symptoms	
Frontal lobe	20	10	0	30
Motor area and Fissura Sylvii	15	8	3	26
Temporal lobe	9	4	2	15
Parietal lobe	10	8	2	20
Occipital lobe	10	4	5	19
Temporo-parieto occipital area	5	2	0	7
Posterior fossa	2	0	0	2

AVM and 12 deeply located AVM. Twelve patients had other types of onset: 8 of them had superficially located AVM and 4 deeply located AVM.

Analysis of the relationship between type of onset and AVM-size showed that 9 of the 71 patients who presented with SAH had large

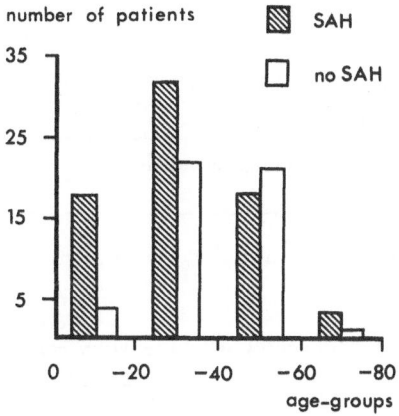

Fig. 26. Distribution of "SAH" and "No-SAH" diagnoses at onset, versus age

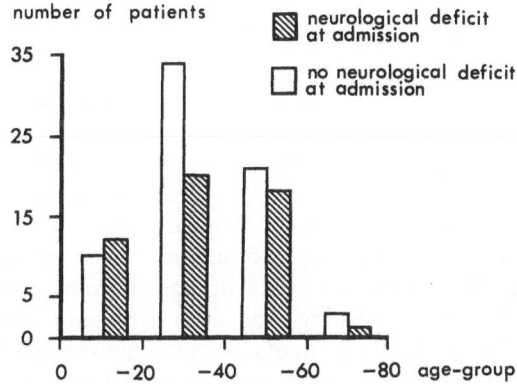

Fig. 27. Distribution of neurological findings at admission, versus age

AVM and 62 had small AVM (13 and 87%, respectively). In the 48 patients with non-SAH onset, the malformation was large in 9 cases and small in 39 cases (19 and 81%, respectively).

Type of onset versus neurology at admission: Of the 71 patients with SAH-onset, 37 had no neurological deficits at admission (52%) and 34 had neurological deficits (48%). Seven of these 34 patients with neurological deficits were comatose and 4 were somnolent (Table 11). Thirty-six patients had an epileptic onset. Twenty-six of them had no neurological symptoms at admission (72%), while 10 had neurological deficits (28%). No patient in the epileptic group was comatose at admission. Of the 12 patients with other types of onset, 5 had no neurological symptoms at admission (42%) and 7 had neurological deficits (58%).

Table 11. *Relationships Between Symptoms at Onset and Neurological Findings at Admission*

Symptoms at onset	Neurological findings at admission
71 SAH	37 pts. without neurol. deficit (1 ICH)
	34 pts. with neurol. deficit — 11 — 4 drowsy / 7 comatose (3 ICH) / 23 focal neurol. deficit (13 ICH)
36 epilepsy	26 pts. without neurol. deficit
	10 pts. with neurol. deficit
12 other symptoms	5 pts. without neurol. deficit
	7 pts. with neurol. deficit

Neurology at admission versus age and sex: 65% of the patients without neurological symptoms at admission were aged below 40 years and 35% were aged above 40 years (Fig. 27). Of the patients with neurological deficits at admission, 63% were aged below 40 years and 37% were 40 years of age or more. Analysis of the relationship between neurology at admission and the patient's sex showed that 35 of the 68 patients without neurological symptoms at admission were women and 33 were men. Of the 51 patients with neurological deficits at admission, 18 were women and 33 men.

Neurology at admission versus AVM-locations and AVM-size: In the 68 patients without neurological symptoms at admission, the malformation was superficially located in 44 and deeply located in 24. Nineteen patients had malformations in the frontal lobe, 8 in the motor region or Sylvian fissure, 7 in the temporal lobe, 12 in the parietal lobe, 6 in the temporo-parieto-occipital lobe, 14 in the occipital area and 2 in the posterior fossa. In the 51 patients with neurological deficits at admission, the malformation was superficially located in 30 and deeply located in 21. Eleven patients had AVM in the frontal lobe, 18 in the motor region or Sylvian fissure, 8 in the temporal lobe, 8 in the parietal lobe, 1 in the temporo-parieto-occipital lobe, and 5 in the occipital area. Analysis of the neurological findings at admission in relation to AVM-size showed that 7 out of 68 patients without neurological symptoms at admission had large AVM while 61 had small AVM (10 and 90%, respectively). Of the 51 patients with neurological deficits at admission, 11 had large AVM and 40 had small AVM (22 and 78%, respectively).

Outcome

As in Chapter IV, the long-term results are presented in relation to both neurological findings and ability to work (Table 12). The patients have been divided into two groups with respect to neurological findings at long-term controls: patients with no or slight neurological symptoms and patients with moderate or severe neurological symptoms. Of the 68 patients without neurological symptoms preoperatively, 58 remained free from symptoms after the operation and are therefore included in the group with no or slight neurological symptoms. Of the 10 remaining patients, 6 died and 4 developed moderate or severe neurological symptoms. Fifty-one patients had neurological deficits preoperatively. Twenty-seven of them were improved after the operation and are included in the group with no or slight neurological symptoms. Ten of the remaining 24 patients died and 14 had persistent neurological deficits or more severe neurological deficits and are included in the group with moderate or severe neurological symptoms. The final analysis of the long-term results in terms of neurological findings showed that 85 patients (72%) had no or slight neurological symptoms. Of the remaining 34 patients (28%), 18 (15%) had moderate or severe neurological symptoms and 16 (13%) died. The symptoms in the 18 patients in the group with moderate or severe neurological symptoms are shown in Table 13.

The patients with epilepsy pre- or postoperatively merit special comment. Of 36 patients with epilepsy as the only preoperative symptom, 31 became well, while in 5 cases the epilepsy was not influenced by the operation. Of 83 operated patients who did not have epilepsy preoperatively, 6 developed epilepsy after the operation.

Analysis of the long-term results with respect to ability to work, showed that 74 out of 85 patients with no or slight neurological symptoms were able to work (87%), while eleven were receiving

Table 12. *Relationships Between Neurological Findings Before Operation and Long-Term Results After Operation*

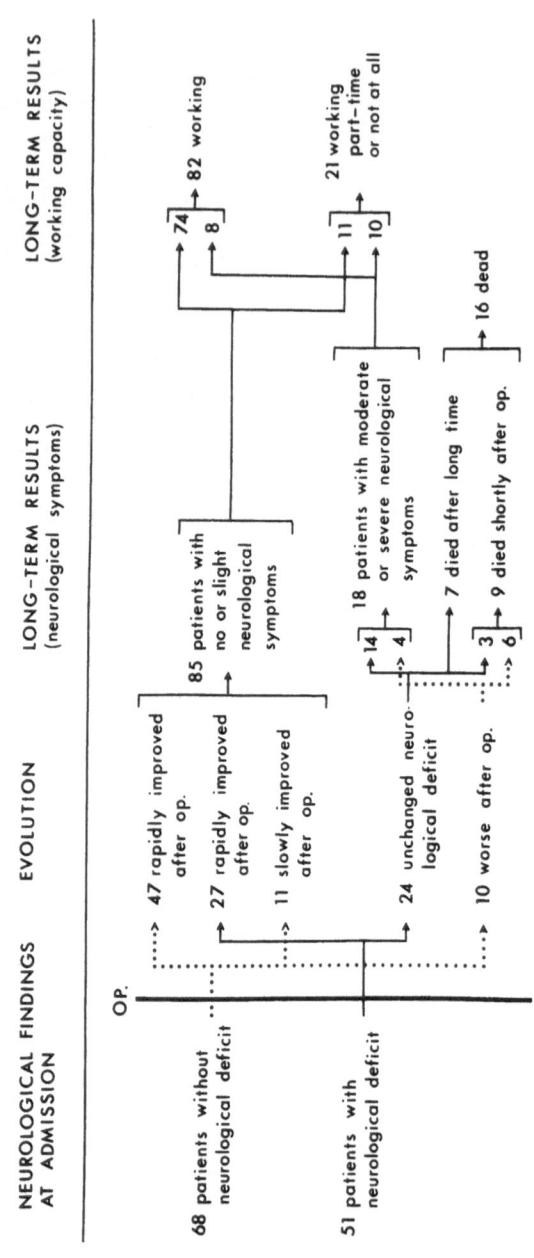

disability pensions or only working part-time (13%). Of the patients with moderate or severe neurological deficits, 8 were working and 10 were not (44 and 56%, respectively). Altogether, 82 patients were thus working full-time and 21 were working only part-time or not at all.

Table 13. *Distribution of Various Sequelae in 18 Operated Patients*

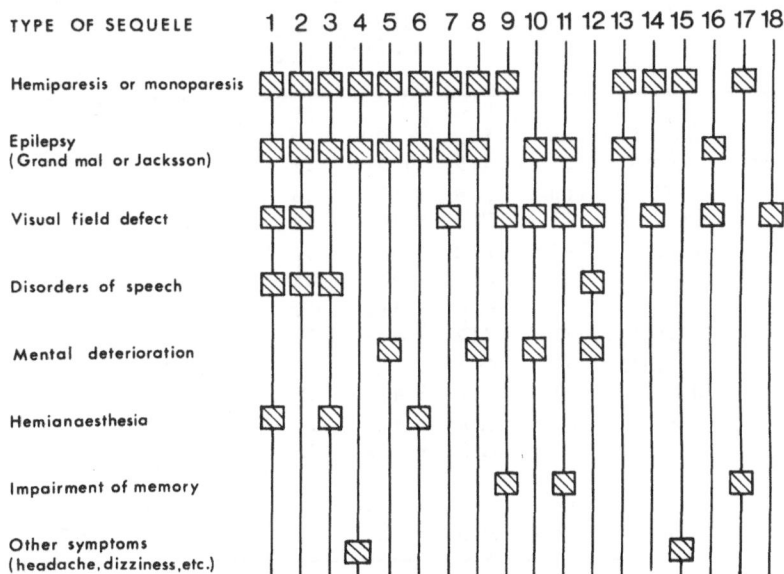

Ranking of Variables

When the long-term results are related to the variables age, sex, AVM-locations and AVM-size, type of onset and neurology at admission, the variables covary differently with the results (Table 14 a). The variables were graded according to their prognostic significance for the final results, as in Chapter IV. One finds that for a patient to have the best chance of being allocated to the group with no or slight neurological symptoms, he should above all be free from neurological deficits at admission. The next most important factor is age below 40 years, and so on (Table 14 b). The patients who are most likely to be allocated to the group with moderate or severe neurological symptoms, on the other hand, exhibit the opposite poles of the same variables, *i.e.*, they had neurological deficits at admission, were aged above 40 years and so on. As was the case for conservatively treated patients, there are also a number of intermediate risk profiles with a more or less favourable prognosis for surgery, depending on the composition.

Table 14 a. *Relationships Between Percentages of Good and Poor Results and Different Variables (Placed in Order of Per Cent Differences) in the Follow-Up of 119 Operated Patients (Each Variable is Devided in Two Poles)*

Long-term results					Moderate or severe neurol. symptoms		Value of significance	Level of significance	Difference in percentage units
Variables	No or slight neurological symptoms								
		No. of cases	%	Difference in %	No. of cases	%			
Neurology at admission	no deficit	58	85.2	+ 70.4	10	14.8	8.08	***	
	deficit	27	52.9	+ 5.8	24	47.1	0	0	64.6
Age	< 40	60	78.9	+ 57.8	16	21.1	6.21	***	
	> 40	25	58.2	+ 16.4	18	41.8	0	0	41.4
Sex	female	42	79.2	+ 58.4	11	20.8	5.18	***	
	male	43	65.1	+ 30.2	23	34.9	2.55	*	28.2
Size	large AVM	12	66.6	+ 33.2	6	33.4	0	0	
	small AVM	73	72.2	+ 44.4	28	27.8	5.16	***	11.2
Symptoms at onset	no SAH	33	68.7	+ 37.4	15	31.3	2.85	**	
	SAH	52	73.2	+ 46.4	19	26.8	4.36	***	9.0
AVM-location	deep	31	68.8	+ 37.6	14	31.2	2.83	**	
	superficial	54	72.9	+ 45.8	20	27.1	4.46	***	8.2
AVM-location	non-silent area	18	69.2	+ 38.4	8	30.8	2.09	*	
	silent area	67	72.0	+ 44.0	26	28.0	4.73	***	5.6

     * 0.01 < p < 0.05.
    ** 0.001 < p < 0.01.
   *** p < 0.001.

Table 14 b. *Most Favourable and Most Unfavourable Risk Profile for Good Results (Operated Patients)*

Graded variables	Polarity favourable for good results	Polarity unfavourable for good results
1—Neurology at admission	= no neurological deficit	— neurological deficit
2—Age at admission	= < 40	— > 40
3—Sex	= female	— male
4—AVM-size	= small	— large
5—Symptoms at onset	= SAH	— no SAH
6—AVM-location	= superficial	— deep
7—AVM-location	= silent area	— nonsilent area

Comparison Between Congruent Risk Profiles in the Nonoperated and Operated Group

Risk profiles have been constructed for all patients in both the surgically treated and conservatively treated group. The polarity for each individual variable was found to point consistently in the same direction for both groups. In other words, age below 40 years meant a good prognosis in both the surgically and the conservatively treated

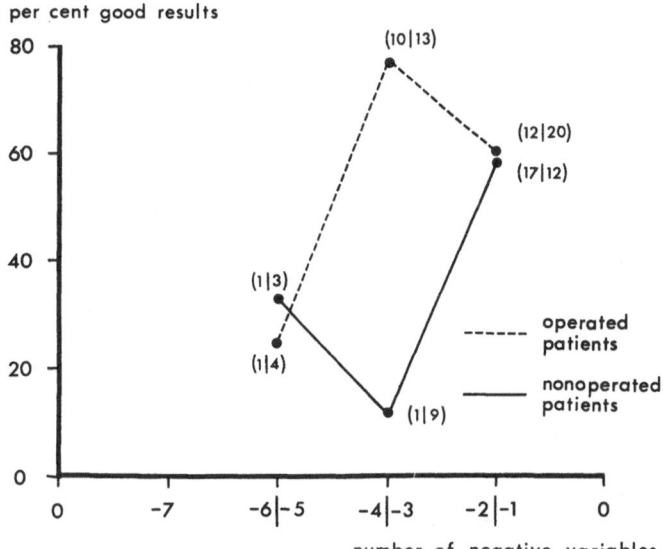

Fig. 28. Relationships between percentages of good results ("no or slight neurological symptoms") and number of negative variables in operated and nonoperated patients having "congruents risk profiles"

group, and so on. The polarity of each variable can therefore be assigned a plus sign or a minus sign, depending on its influence on the prognosis, regardless of the method of treatment.

There is no doubt, however, that the variables have different prognostic value. Comparisons between the operated and non-operated group can therefore not be based on simple summation of variables. The comparison will only be valid when patients with identical profiles are compared, *i.e.*, patients whose polarity in + and — for the same variables coincides. These risk profiles may be described as *congruent*.

Patients with congruent risk profiles may be considered identical up until the decision whether or not to operate. These congruent risk

profiles may therefore be used for comparison of the results in the
two groups. This is illustrated in Fig. 28. The y-axis shows the
number of restituted patients in percent of the total number of
patients in each treatment group. The x-axis shows the risk profiles
grouped on a scale from — 7 to 0. Zero represents a patient without
negative variables, who thus has 7 positive variables in the same
congruent risk profile. Similarly, — 3 represents 3 negative and
4 positive variables. Our series of congruent risk profiles (61 patients)
includes no representatives of the extreme positions zero and — 7.
Since the number of congruent profiles is small, the risk profiles have
been combined into three groups, representing the values — 1 — 2,
— 3 — 4, and — 5 — 6. It will be seen from the figure that
congruent risk profiles belonging to the group — 1 — 2 and the
group — 5 — 6 show no significant difference in results between
operated and nonoperated patients. For the group — 3 — 4, however, there is a significant difference ($p < 0.01$) in favour of the
operated patients.

Discussion

The relationships between the seven variables of the operated
patient do not differ markedly from the relationships between the
same variables described in Chapter IV concerning the natural
history of patients with AVM. The material as a whole is, however,
selected according to the criteria of operability described in
Chapter III.

The group of operated patients includes probably more high-risk
patients than the conservatively treated group, since patients with
SAH were given priority for surgery. The groups are thus not
identical and direct comparison between the groups as a whole is
therefore not valid. By comparing patients with congruent risk
profiles in the two groups, our method reduces the influence of this
source of error.

There is a certain difference between the ranking of the variables
according to the surgeon's original selection of patients for surgery
and the ranking of variables with knowledge of the long-term results.
In the ranking according to the long-term results, patient variables,
such as neurology at admission, age and sex, are given a more
prominent place than in the original selection. It may be concluded
that the surgeon based his decision mainly on the operability of the
AVM, AVM-size, and AVM-location being the most important
factors. He also considered the type of onset, giving priority to
patients with SAH-onset, but attached less importance to patient
variables. In no case, for example, did the clinician state the patient's

sex as the reason for the decision for or against surgery. The fact that this variable nevertheless has a prominent place in the context of the long-term results may be due to the sex variable covarying with other variables. It cannot be excluded, however, that the sex variable *per se* is important. Sex is known to be of importance in other medical contexts, women having been shown to have a better restitutional capacity than men [36].

Of the 119 patients who were subjected to surgery, 16 died. Detailed analysis of the causes of death showed that only 6 of the deaths could be directly related to the operation: three of these patients died from uncontrollable haemorrhage during the operation and three from postoperative haematoma. Three patients were comatose at admission and died postoperatively. In the latter three cases there is reason to conclude that the outcome would have been the same without surgery. Three patients died long after the operation from recurrence of haemorrhage from partially extirpated AVM. These deaths can probably be attributed to the natural history of AVM, regardless of whether or not surgery is performed. On the other hand, it is possible that partial extirpation might have altered the haemodynamics in such a way as to favour recurrence of haemorrhage. The remaining 4 patients died from other causes, although one of these deaths may have been due to recurrence of haemorrhage (cerebrovascular insult).

The operative mortality, with the above reservations, was thus 5.0% (6 out of 119). This figure may be compared with the mortality in the nonoperated patients, of whom 6.4% died from primary haemorrhage and 12.5% from recurrence of haemorrhage. It is, of course, not known whether any of the patients who died from primary haemorrhage could have been saved by operation. If these early deaths are excluded, the 12.5% of the patients who died from recurrence of haemorrhage may be compared with the 5.0% who died in connection with the operation. It might thus be argued that the risk of death in the nonoperated group is 2.5 (12.5/5) times greater than in the operated group.

The morbidity also favours surgery. Of the survivors in the operated group, 95 patients (83%) had no or slight neurological symptoms, while 18 (17%) had moderate or severe neurological symptoms. Of the survivors in the nonoperated group, 43% had no or slight neurological symptoms while 57% had moderate or severe neurological symptoms. The question is, is this obvious difference in morbidity due to the original selection or to the operation as such, regardless of selection?

Patients with good results were found to have similar risk profiles in both the operated and the nonoperated group. The percentage of favourable risk profiles was, however, highest in the operated group and the percentage of unfavourable risk profiles was highest in the nonoperated group. This suggests that the selection influenced the results, which means that the groups as a whole cannot be compared. When the results for congruent risk profiles in the two groups are compared, however, one finds equally good results with both methods of treatment in patients with markedly favourable or markedly unfavourable risk profiles. In an intermediate group, in which the risk profiles contain approximately equally many favourable and unfavourable variables, the results were significantly better in the operated group. From this finding it may be concluded that surgery is generally to be preferred to conservative treatment. This conclusion is based on a relatively small number of patients, however. The problem will be further discussed in Chapter VI, where the profile variables are weighed and graded so that the risk profiles have a more differentiated numerical value. This means that a very much larger number of numerically equal risk profiles than congruent risk profiles in the operated and nonoperated group may be compared with each other and evaluated with statistical methods.

Assessment of the results of treatment of patients with AVM must thus be based on the total results, *i.e.*, it must include both operated and nonoperated patients. If only the operated group is considered and one asks whether the results can be improved, the answer will obviously be "yes". It is quite clear that the results in the operated group will be better if only patients with favourable risk profiles are operated upon and only the results in operated patients are presented. It must then be borne in mind that patients whose risk profiles are less favourable or unfavourable for both methods of treatment will then be allocated to the nonoperated group. Our study indicates that although this transfer will lead to better results of surgery, the overall results will be poorer. It therefore follows that comparisons between different operated series are unreliable since the results depend on the selection criteria, although the surgical technique used and the surgeon's skill may be of marginal importance.

VI. The Decision Process and Assessment of the Prognosis

Luigi Pellettieri, Carl-Axel Carlsson, and Sven Grevsten [*]

Introduction

It has been shown in Chapters IV and V that several patient-AVM constellations (risk profiles) which give good and poor results are similar in the operated and the nonoperated group. It has previously been reported [52] that operable patients have a favourable prognosis even without operation and this finding has been used as an argument in support of conservative treatment. Our study has shown that this conclusion is not correct as we found a higher frequency of good results for congruent risk profiles in the operated group. We therefore conclude that surgical treatment of AVM is probably to be preferred to conservative treatment. This conclusion is drawn with certain reservations, however, as for parts of the risk-profile scale there are only a few patients with congruent risk profiles, where a comparison is possible. Only in one of the three subgroups of measurement there is a significant difference in treatment results in favour of the operated group ($p < 0.01$), while in the other two there is no difference (see Fig. 28, Chapter V).

In this analysis we have endeavoured to increase the possibilities of evaluation by quantifying the profile variables and giving each individual risk profile a numerical value (expressed as the sum of the variables). This yields larger groups of risk profiles with the same value. The creation of these data increases the possibilities of carrying out an adequate analysis of the AVM material.

Patients and Methods

The study comprises 166 consecutive cases of intracranial AVM investigated and treated at the Department of Neurosurgery at Sahlgren Hospital in Gothenburg between 1953 and 1971. The patients have been described in Chapters II, III, IV, and V.

[*] Department of General Surgery, Academic Hospital, University of Uppsala, Uppsala, Sweden.

Methods of Calculation

General principles: To enable readers to follow the mathematical analysis of the results of treatment, the method will be presented and discussed in some detail.

The following expression is a mathematical transformation of the clinical variables:

$$X_1; X_2; X_3; \ldots; X_n \tag{1}$$

Each variable X_i where ($i = 1, 2, 3, \ldots, n$) represents a clinical variable used for guidance when deciding on the treatment. The variable X_i acquires positive value when the clinical information is prognostically favourable and negative value when the information is prognostically unfavourable. For example, age below 40 years means a positive prognosis and the variable is given a positive value. Age above 40 years means a negative prognosis and the variable is given a negative value. The variables X_i can have differing prognostic value. Thus, the variables

$$X_1; X_2; X_3; \ldots, X_{n_1} \tag{2}$$
$$(n_1 < n)$$

may have greater prognostic value than the variables

$$X_{n_1 + 1}; X_{n_1 + 2}; X_{n_1 + 3}; \ldots; X_{n_2}, \tag{3}$$
$$(n_2 < n)$$

which in turn have greater prognostic value than the variables

$$X_{n_2 + 1}; X_{n_2 + 2}; X_{n_2 + 3}; \ldots; X_{n_3}, \tag{4}$$
$$(n_3 < n)$$

In expressions 2, 3, and 4

$$n_1 + n_2 + n_3 + \ldots = n \tag{5}$$

The calculated prognostic values of the variables: In our patients we have identified 7 variables that are important for a correct judgement of the prognosis. The prognostic value of a single variable compared to other variables is estimated from the extent to which the variable covaries with the results of treatment in the two groups, operated and nonoperated patients.

In the medical context, precise figures are usually inadequate for grading clinical variables which differ in "character". This also applies to the variables occurring in our patients (age, sex, symptoms at onset, neurology at admission, AVM-size and AVM-location). This heterogeneity between the variables makes a descriptive statistical analysis necessary. We have therefore graded each decision variable X_i in terms of pluses and minuses ($+$, $++$, $+++$, $++++/$ $-$, $--$, $---$, $----$), depending on the prognosis and the amount of prognostic information which each variable contains according to different guiding tests (chi-square test and Fisher's test for the comparison of two proportions) as well as the estimated covariance between each variable and the final result of the treatment.

The estimated symbolic values of the variables: Using the method described above, the 7 variables which together constitute the risk profile in both operated and nonoperated patients may be expressed in symbolic relative figures which indicate the prognostic value of the variables. The procedure can be illustrated with an example: In the nonoperated group (Table 8 a, Chapter IV) 50% of the patients aged below 40 years have moderate or severe neurological symptoms, while 50% have no or slight neurological symptoms. The difference is 50–50% = 0%. In the age-group above 40 years 80% have moderate or severe neurological symptoms and 20% no or slight neurological symptoms. The difference is 80–20% = 60%. The difference between these two differences, expressed in percentage units (0–60% = 60%) may be regarded as a symbolic relative measure of the prognostic value of the age variable in favour of patients below 40 years of age. The corresponding calculation for the variable "neurology at admission" gives a difference of 52 percentage units in favour of patients with normal neurology at admission compared to patients admitted with a neurological deficit. Comparison between these variables thus shows that the age variable is of greater prognostic value than the variable "neurology at admission", expressed in percentage units (60% compared to 52%). The prognostic value of the other variables can be evaluated in percentage units and weighed against one another in an analogous way.

The above procedure was applied to the operated and the nonoperated group and the variables were then symbolically graded in each group separately from $+$ to $++++$ and $-$ to $----$, the positive sign being used to evaluate the variable's prognostically favourable polarization and the negative sign to evaluate its prognostically unfavourable polarization (Table 16).

This symbolic grading was carried out in the following way: Since the highest value is about 60 percentage units, each point on a four-point scale represents about 15 percentage units. The scale limits were thus set at 15, 30, and 45 percentage units. Further for each variable the symbolic values for the two treatment groups were then added together and divided by 2 (and rounded off upwards to the nearest whole number where necessary) so as to give a mean value for the information from the two groups (Table 16).

The calculated risk profile: Finally, the net total of the pluses and minuses from the different variables was calculated for each patient, as follows:

$$X_1 + X_2 + X_3 + X_4 + \ldots + X_n = \sum_{i=1}^{n} X_i \qquad (6)$$

This gives the "risk profile" for each patient.

In our patients the summation of the symbolic values of the variables in a single risk profile gave a maximum of 16 plus signs or 16 minus signs.

These totals, representing individual risk profiles, were related to the final results of the treatment. Patients with similar "risk profiles" in the two treatment groups could then be compared.

Results

Calculated prognostic values of the variables: The analysis of the prognostic value of different variables in the nonoperated and operated groups showed that the positive pole of each variable co-varied equally and consistently with a positive prognosis in both groups. For example, the pole below 40 years in the age variable is associated with a better prognosis than the pole "above 40 years" in both the nonoperated and the operated group. This has been checked for the whole material with Fisher's test (see Table 8 a, Chapter IV, and Table 14 a, Chapter V, where the significance values are given). The χ^2 test has been used to determine the prognostic value of each variable in the two treatment groups separately. This analysis shows that neurology at admission and age are the only variables which show a significant covariance with the results in both treatment groups. This indicates that these two variables are of greater prognostic value than the other variables (for neurology at admission $p < 0.05$ in the nonoperated group and $p < 0.001$ in the operated group: for age $p < 0.05$ in both groups). The χ^2 test was also used to check the prognostic significance of each individual variable for surgery and conservative treatment (Table 15). The outcome was consistently better for surgery.

The estimated symbolic values of the variables: Table 16 shows the estimated symbolic values for each variable in the operated and nonoperated group and the calculated symbolic mean values. This symbolic mean value constitutes the prognostic value of the variable, which is used to calculate the value of each individual patient's

Table 15. χ^2-test on "Isolated Variables", Showing the Significance of Better Results With Operation, for Each Variable, in Comparison With Conservative Treatment

Variables	Value of significance	Level of significance
No deficit at admission	10.18	**
Deficit at admission	6.24	*
Age < 40 at admission	7.38	**
Age > 40 at admission	10.1	**
AVM-location, superficial	5.52	*
AVM-location, deep	11.95	***
AVM-location, silent area	11.45	***
AVM-location, nonsilent area	9.14	**
Sex female	7.27	**
Sex male	13.76	***
AVM-size, small	9.31	**
AVM-size, large	6.51	*
SAH at onset	10.13	**
No SAH at onset	6.98	**

   * $0.01 < p < 0.05$.
  ** $0.001 < p < 0.01$.
 *** $p < 0.001$.

risk profile. The table only shows the two most extreme risk profiles on the risk-profile scale: the one for the most positive and the one for the most negative results. Between these two extreme risk profiles there are, in our material, a large number (160) of intermediate risk profiles with more or less good prognostic value, depending on the combinations of variables. Theoretically, 128 different types of risk profile are possible. We found 85 different types in our patients.

The calculated risk profiles: The long-term results in subgroups with numerically equivalent risk profiles calculated according to the previously described method in the operated and nonoperated groups are compared in Fig. 29. The x-axis shows the symbolic value of the risk profiles and the y-axis the percentage of patients in the total material who had no or slight neurological symptoms in each risk-profile group in the long-term results. Note that the total material includes patients who died. The diagram shows that the treatment results were consistently better in patients who were operated upon than in those who were not. The difference is marked for the risk profiles in the middle of the risk scale. Significant differences ($p < 0.01$) in results were found in this part of the scale (between — 2 and + 2 on the risk-profile scale).

Table 16. *Calculation of Symbolic Prognostic Values for the 7 Variables*

Bipolarly classified variables	Nonoperated patients		Operated patients		Sum of symbolic values	Final grading	Long-termed results	
	Differences in percent	Symbolic values	Differences in percent	Symbolic values			Good	Poor
Neurology at admission (no deficit/deficit)	52.0%	= 4	64.6%	= 4	8	4	no deficit = + 4	deficit = − 4
Age at admission (< 40/> 40)	60.0%	= 4	41.4%	= 3	7	4	< 40 = + 4	> 40 = − 4
AVM-location (superficial/deep)	40.0%	= 3	8.2%	= 1	4	2	superficial = + 2	deep = − 2
AVM-location (silent/nonsilent)	38.8%	= 3	5.6%	= 1	4	2	silent area = + 2	nonsil. area = − 2
Sex (female/male)	10.1%	= 1	28.2%	= 2	3	2	female = + 2	male = − 2
AVM-size (small/large)	12.4%	= 1	11.2%	= 1	2	1	small = + 1	large = − 1
Symptoms at onset (SAH/no SAH)	0.6%	= 1	9.0%	= 1	2	1	SAH = + 1	no SAH = − 1

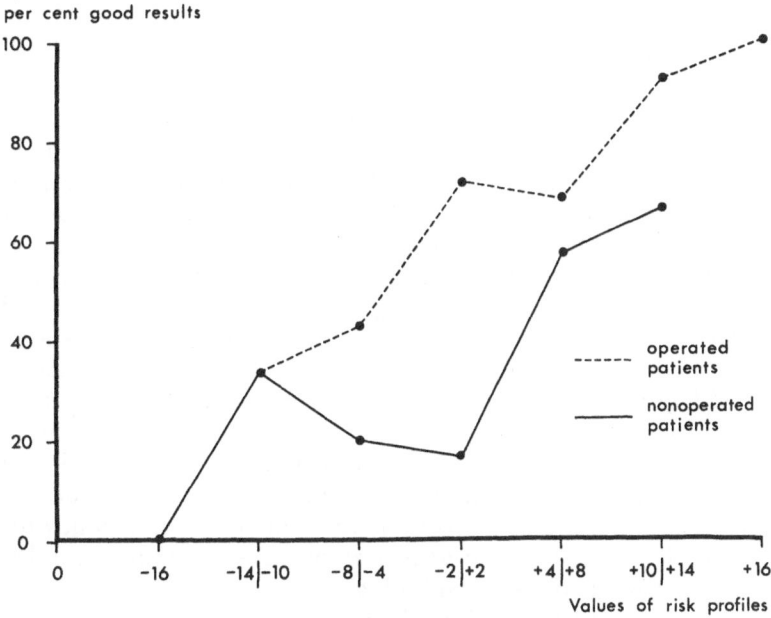

per cent good results

Fig. 29. Diagram illustrating the relationships between values of the risk profiles and percentages good results in the two treatment groups

Discussion

We have already declared (Chapter III) that when analysing a clinical decision it is important to identify which clinical variables, among all possible, have formed the basis of the therapeutic decision. According to the case records, the judgement was based on seven main variables. One of these variables is sex, which we found important for judging the prognosis but which was not used by the surgeon in connection with his original selection. The analysis has been limited to these seven variables, although it would theoretically have been possible to increase the amount of information. Studies have shown that, beyond a certain limit, the quality of the decision does not increase with the amount of information available. In medical decision-making, about five variables generally give the best performance [30, 47].

Our aim was to rate these seven variables in such a way as to define their prognostic significance for the final results. In order to do this, we had to study the covariance of each individual variable with the results. The reliability of this rating is undermined by the inevitable interaction between the variables (see Discussion in Chapter III). It is almost impossible to analyse the degree of interaction mathematically, owing to the differing "character" of the variables. An analysis of the "isolated" variables gives the best possible clinical rating of the treatment prognosis.

The prognostic value of the variables has been studied by means of Fisher's test and the χ^2 test. It must be emphasized that the small number of patients in the nonoperated group limits the representativeness of the tests for this group of patients. The combined information yielded by these tests shows that the variables have different prognostic value. The results of the significance tests form a basis for rating the variables. The percentage differences between the variables in relation to the results, translated into symbolic values, provide a simple method of rating the variables in the nonoperated and the operated group. Summation of the symbolic values from the two groups, variable by variable, gives mean values which can be used for final rating of the variables. This summation of symbolic values is possible since the variables have the same "polarity" in both treatment groups, *i.e.*, for each variable, the same pole corresponds to the same results in both treatment groups. For example, age below 40 years means good results in both groups.

The risk profiles constructed from the symbolic mean values of the variables may seem oversimplified as each variable included in the risk profile was given only two poles, with no possibility of detailed variation for the individual patient. The symbolic risk value of the variables in plus and minus points is only intended for use when rating the variables in relation to one another. Further variations in the individual variable—ages above and below 40 years, AVM-sizes below and above 3 cm, etc.—have already been considered in the bipolar definition. A more precise differentiation of the variables has previously been tested and was found not to be useful for comparison between the variables.

The diagram in Fig. 29 expresses the relationship between numerically equivalent risk profiles and long-term results in the two treatment groups. It will be seen that the results are better in the operated than in the nonoperated patients for risk groups in the middle of the risk-profile scale. The conclusion drawn in Chapters IV and V and presented in the introduction to this chapter are thus confirmed. They can be formulated as follows: the long-term results for the extremes of the risk-profile scale in the two treatment groups were more dependent on the composition of the risk profile and less influenced by the type of treatment—surgery or conservative treatment. In the middle of the scale, however, the results show a statistically significant difference ($p < 0.01$) in favour of surgery in this relatively large group of patients. Analysis of the prognostic value of individual variables (see results of the χ^2 test in Table 1) shows consistently better results in the operated group.

The diagram in Fig. 29 shows how the individual variables interact so that the central subgroup of patients benefits more by operation. The diagram may be used for prognostic assessment of the individual AVM patient. The different variables for the patient are assigned plus or minus signs, in accordance with Table 16, and simple summation gives the total score for the risk profile. The prognosis for surgery and conservative treatment can then be read off directly from the diagram in Fig. 29. The diagram can therefore be used for assessment of the prognosis when deciding whether or not to operate in the individual case. It must be remembered, however, that occasional patients may deviate from the normal pattern.

If the risk-profile value is low (— 10 or below on the risk-profile scale) the prognosis is equally poor with surgery and conservative treatment. From — 8 and upwards on the scale there is a clear tendency for surgery to give better results, and from — 2 to + 2 this tendency is statistically significant ($p < 0.01$).

In patients with an unfavourable combination of variables other methods of treatment may be preferable, e.g., artificial embolization or X-ray irradiation of the AVM. In borderline cases on the minus range of the risk-profile scale, the observation (see Chapter II) that the presence of the back flow phenomenon on the angiogram means less risk of haemorrhage may be of help in the decision.

For all patients with a favourable combination of variables the indications for operation become stronger if the time dimension is considered. With the passage of time, a patient who had a certain score at the moment of decision will show a shift towards a lower score on the risk-profile scale as he or she grows older, the malformation may grow and the patient's neurological condition may deteriorate owing to new haemorrhages. This means that the prognosis becomes poorer with time.

The appearance of the diagram may partly explain the extreme attitudes in the "surgery versus conservative treatment" dispute, reflected in the literature [23, 52]. The authors who have been confronted with patients who, in our study, would have been found in the middle of the risk-profile scale have been convinced that surgery is the most effective mode of therapy. The authors who advocate conservative treatment, on the other hand, have probably mainly considered patients belonging to the risk groups at the extreme minus or plus end of the scale. In these groups the difference in favour of surgery is not significant.

VII. General Discussion and Conclusion

Luigi Pellettieri

A treatment programme is the result of deliberation in which the therapist weighs a number of different factors against one another. In his efforts to exert maximum control over the course of the disease, he assesses not only the relevant facts as they present themselves at that moment but also the likely future course. Each symptom or item of information is thus assigned both spatial and temporal dimensions. Different factors (symptoms or data) are assigned differing importance, depending on their relative magnitude and rate of change with time. Certain factors are directly related to the disease itself, while others are related to the patient who has the disease. There are also other factors which are not directly related to the patient or to the disease. All these factors may influence the decision-maker, including the latter factors, which may be termed "external circumstances" and include such factors as the patient's attitude to his disease and to different types of treatment. A patient with AVM may be unable to face the thought of living with this threat and may insist on having an operation even if the surgeon is doubtful, while another patient may refuse surgery and nullify the surgeon's decision to operate. The surgeon himself is, of course, another variable and fluctuations of mood may influence his decision.

In theory, an adequate decision should be based on all the factors involved in the process one wishes to influence. This, in turn, presupposes that one knows how much importance to attach to different factors when reaching a decision. Both these conditions are in practice very difficult to fulfil. Each clinician develops his own method of evaluating which factors are of importance, based on personal experience. He will also attribute different importance to different factors. This assignment of higher priority to certain factors means that factors considered to have little or no importance will gradually be excluded from the assessment.

As AVM is a relatively uncommon disease, the individual surgeon's experience will be limited and his ranking of different factors in order of importance may be erroneous. He may overrate the importance of factors which support his own views on how to treat the disease and neglect factors which do not. The clinician may also draw the wrong parallels. For example, he may unconsciously tend to compare AVM with arterial aneurysms and favour surgery because he overrates the risk of haemorrhage. On the other hand, the clinician may have developed a conservative attitude towards the disease in general, particularly when surgical treatment does not give unequivocally better results.

In this study, which is a statistical analysis of the results of surgery and conservative treatment in AVM-patients, the different factors used in the decision process have been called "variables". Together, these variables make up the "risk profile". The risk profile thus describes relevant characteristics of the patient and his malformation. The synonymous designation "patient-AVM constellations" has therefore also been used at times.

Both the number of variables and their identification was based on information given by the clinician in the case records. In this context it is obviously an advantage that all the patients were treated at the same clinic, so that the selection criteria for surgery or conservative treatment were fairly uniform.

The number of variables making up the risk profiles have been carefully considered. We were forced to strike a balance between the wish to include as many variables as possible, in order to make the study complete, and the need to limit their number, owing to the relatively small number of patients. These methodological problems should be seen as an indication that the prognostic implications and treatment policy proposed should be applied with certain reservations.

The main purpose of this study was to draw up guidelines for treatment of patients with AVM, *i.e.*, for the decision between surgery and conservative treatment. It is quite clear that this problem cannot be resolved by comparing the overall results in different groups of operated and nonoperated patients. The original selection means that the groups are not directly comparable. In this study patients with equivalent risk profiles in each group were therefore compared. The study comprises a consecutive series of 166 patients treated at the Department of Neurosurgery at Sahlgren Hospital, Gothenburg, between 1953 and 1971. 119 were subjected to surgery and 47 were given conservative treatment. A detailed description of the patients is given in Chapter II. The vascularization, location, and size of the malformations are presented in relation to the patient's age and sex. The variables that formed the basis of the decision whether or not to operate have been identified (Chapter III). Seven variables were found to be most important: neurology at admission, the patient's age and sex, symptoms at onset, AVM-size, AVM-deeply or superficially located, and AVM-location in silent or nonsilent areas. The sex variable was not used by the surgeon in his original treatment decision. This variable was introduced retrospectively as it proved to be important for the results. The variables were subsequently used for analysis of the conservatively (Chapter IV) and surgically (Chapter V) treated patients. The extent to which the variables covaried with the long-term treatment results was calculated using a special method. Based on this calculation, a specific prognostic risk profile was constructed for each patient.

We found a limited number of congruent risk profiles in the two treatment groups. Comparison between these groups indicated that surgery generally seems to give better results than conservative treatment (Chapter V). In Chapter VI the variables were assigned numerical values, calculated from the results, in order to be able to make a more detailed judgement. Positive values symbolize favourable results and negative values unfavourable results. The variables included in the risk profile were then totalled so as to give a numerical value for each risk profile. These values were used to group the risk profiles on a scale from the most favourable to the most unfavourable, with extreme values of $+16$ and -16. This method results in a number of risk profiles with the same numerical value in both treatment groups and thus allows comparisons over a large part of the risk-profile scale. This comparison is illustrated in Fig. 29, in Chapter VI.

We found that low risk-profile values (-10 or below) were associated with a poor prognosis in both groups. At values of -8 and above on the risk-profile scale surgery tended to give consistently better results. Within the segment $-2 + 2$ surgery gave significantly better results ($p < 0.01$).

From these findings it may be concluded that surgical treatment is indicated in most patients with AVM. Conservative treatment may be justifiable in the worst patients (those with scores below -10 on the risk-profile scale), however, since the type of treatment does not seem to influence the outcome in these patients.

This method can be used for each individual patient with AVM. By assigning numerical values to the variables, as described in Chapter VI, the numerical value of the risk profile can be calculated and the prognosis for surgery and conservative treatment can be estimated.

In our material the clinician's original evaluation of the variables when deciding whether or not to operate can be compared with the evaluation performed with knowledge of the results. This comparison shows fairly good agreement between the two assessments, indicating that the clinician's original decision, based on experience, was correct on the whole. The assessments are not in complete concordance, however. The clinician seems to have overrated the AVM-variables and underrated the patient-variables to some extent. It is possible that surgeons tend to give priority to technical variables relating to the operation. The analysis also showed that the surgeon was not completely consistent in his assessment as equivalent profiles were found in both treatment groups. This was, in fact, a prerequisite for this study. The inconsistency in the assessment may, in some cases, have been due to the influence of uncontrollable variables, such as the patient's attitude to his disease and its treatment. In other cases the inconsistency may have been an expression of the surgeon's ambivalence. He may have weighed an unfavourable variable against a favourable variable and found the balance to be in favour of operation in one case, while in another case he may have decided that the same combination of variables justified a decision against surgery. There may also be subtle differences in the evaluation which could not be detected in our analysis.

Fig. 29 (Chapter VI) seems to offer an explanation for the opposing views on the question of treatment of AVM—conservative treatment versus surgery. It shows that a favourable combination of variables gives relatively good results with both modes of therapy and that the results deteriorate proportionately with falling values on the risk-profile scale in both groups. Although surgery tends to give better results, the difference is only significant within a limited range on the risk-profile scale. The relative concordance between the curves probably explains the controversy between those who advocate surgery and those who prefer conservative treatment.

References

1. Bergstrand, H., Olivecrona, H., Tönnis, W., Gefäßmißbildungen und Gefäß-geschwülste des Gehirns, pp. 181. Leipzig: G. Thieme. 1936.
2. Buche, K.-A., Bockhorn, J., Schäfer, E. R., Macro- and microsurgery of central angiomas. Berlin-Heidelberg-New York: Springer. 1974.
3. Christensen, E., Larsen, H., Fatal subarachnoid haemorrhages in pregnant women with intracranial and intramedullary vascular malformations. Acta psychiat. Scand. 29 (1954), 441.
4. Courville, C. B., Pathology of the nervous system, 2nd ed. Mountain View, Cal.: Pacific Press Publ. Ass. 1945.
5. Cushing, H., Bailey, P., Tumors arising from the blood-vessels of the brain. Angiomatous malformations and hemangioblastomas. Springfield, Ill.: Ch. C Thomas. 1928.
6. Dandy, W. E., Arteriovenous aneurysm of the brain. Arch. Surg. 17 (1928), 190.
7. Dandy, W. E., Venous abnormalities and angiomas of the brain. Arch. Surg. 17 (1928), 715.
8. Evans, N. G., Courville, C. B., Notes on the pathogenesis and morphology of new growths, malformations and deformities of the intracranial blood vessels. Bull. Los Angeles Neurol. Soc. 4 (1939), 145.
9. Forster, M. D., Steiner, L., Håkanson, S., Arteriovenous malformations of the brain. A long-term clinical study. J. Neurosurg. 37 (1972), 562.
10. Gillingham, J., Arteriovenous malformations of the head. Edinb. Med. J. 60 (1953), 305.
11. Hamby, W. B., The pathology of supratentorial angiomas. J. Neurosurg. 15 (1958), 65.
12. Henderson, W. R., Gomez, R. de R. L., Natural history of cerebral angiomas. Brit. Med. J. 4 (1967), 571.
13. Höök, O., Johanson, C., Intracranial arteriovenous aneurysms. A. M. A. Arch. Neurol. Psychiat. 80 (1958), 39.
14. Johnson, R. T., Surgery of cerebral hemorrhage. In: Recent advances in neurology, p. 124 (Lord Brain, Maria Wilkinson, eds.). London: Churchill. 1969.
15. Kaplan, H. A., Aronson, S. M., Browder, E. J., Vascular malformations of the brain. An anatomical study. J. Neurosurg. 18 (1961), 630.
16. Krayenbühl, H., Siebermann, R., Small vascular malformations as a cause of primary intracerebral hemorrhage. J. Neurosurg. 22 (1965), 7.
17. Krayenbühl, H., Yaşargil, M. G., Das Hirnaneurysma. Basel: J. R. Geigy S. A. 1958.
18. Krayenbühl, H., Discussion des rapports sur les angiomes supratentoriels. 1er Congrès International de Neurochirurgie, p. 263. Bruxelles. 1957.
19. Krenchel, N. J., Intracranial racemose angiomas, a clinical study. Aarhus: Universitetsforlaget. 1961.

20. Kunc, Z., Possibility of surgery in arteriovenous malformation in the anatomically important and dangerous regions of the brain. J. Neurol. Neurosurg. Psychiat. 28 (1965), 183.

21. Lange-Cosack, H., Norlén, G., Tönnis, W., Walter, W., Klinik und Behandlung der raumbeengenden intrakraniellen Prozesse. II. In: Handbuch der Neurochirurgie (Olivecrona, H., Tönnis, W., eds.). Berlin-Heidelberg-New York: Springer. 1966.

22. Luessenhop, A. J., Kachmann, R., Shevlin, W., Ferrero, A. A., Clinical evaluation of artificial embolisation in the management of large cerebral arteriovenous malformation. J. Neurosurg. 23 (1965), 400.

23. Luessenhop, A. J., Operative treatment of arteriovenous malformations of the brain. Current controversies in neurosurgery, p. 203 (Morley, T. P., ed.). Philadelphia, Pa.: W. B. Saunders Company. 1976.

24. MacKenzie, I., The clinical presentation of the cerebral angioma. Review of 50 cases. Brain 76 (1953), 184.

25. McCormick, W. F., The pathology of vascular ("arterio-venous") malformations. J. Neurosurg. 24 (1966), 867.

26. McKissock, W., Hankinson, J., The surgical treatment of the supratentorial angiomas. Rapports et discussions. 1er Congrès International de Neurochirurgie, Bruxelles. 1957.

27. Noran, H. H., Intracranial vascular tumors and malformations. Arch. Path. 39 (1945), 393.

28. Norlén, G., Arteriovenous aneurysms of the brain. Report of 10 cases of total removal of lesion. J. Neurosurg. 6 (1949), 475.

29. Norlén, G., Die chirurgische Behandlung von intrakraniellen Gefäßmißbildungen. A. Angiome. In: Handbuch der Neurochirurgie, Vol. IV, p. 146 (Olivecrona, H., Tönnis, W., eds.). Berlin-Heidelberg-New York: Springer. 1966.

30. Nysted, L., Magnusson, D., Predictive efficiency as a function of amount of information. Multivariate Behavioral Research 7 (1972), 441.

31. Nyström, S. H. M., Congenital arteriovenous malformations of the brain. Helsinki, Finland. 1975.

32. Olivecrona, H., Ladenheim, J., Congenital arteriovenous aneurysms of the carotid and vertebral systems. Berlin-Göttingen-Heidelberg: Springer. 1957.

33. Olivecrona, H., Riives, J., Arteriovenous aneurysms of the brain, their diagnosis and treatment. Arch. Neurol. Psychiat. 59 (1948), 567.

34. Padget, D. H., The cranial venous system in man in reference to development, adult configuration, and relation to the arteries. Amer. J. Anat. 98 (1956), 307.

35. Paterson, J. H., McKissock, W., A clinical survey of intracranial angiomas with special reference to their mode of progression and surgical treatment. A report of 110 cases. Brain 79 (1956), 233.

36. Perman, E., Sex differences in morbidity and mortality. Nordisk Medicin 16 (1956), 537.

37. Perret, G. E., Nishioka, H., Report on the cooperative study of intracranial aneurysms and subarachnoid hemorrhage. Arteriovenous malformations. J. Neurosurg. 25 (1966), 467.

38. Pia, H. W., The indications and contraindications for treatment or assessment in cerebral angiomas. Advances in diagnosis and therapy (Pia, H. W., Gleave, I. R. W., Grote, E., Zierski, J., eds.). Berlin-Heidelberg-New York: Springer. 1975.

39. Pia, H. W., The acute treatment of cerebral arteriovenous angiomas associated with hematomas. Berlin-Heidelberg-New York: Springer. 1974.

40. Pool, J. L., Potts, D. G., Aneurysms and arteriovenous anomalies of the brain. New York: Harper & Row. 1965.
41. Porter, A. J., Bull, J., Some aspects of the natural history of cerebral arteriovenous malformation. Brit. J. Radiol. 42 (1969), 667.
42. Potter, J. M., Angiomatous malformations of the brain: their nature and prognosis. Ann. Roy. Coll. Surg. Eng. 16 (1955), 227.
43. Robinson, J. L., Hall, C. S., Sedzimir, C. B., Arteriovenous malformations aneurysms and pregnancy. J. Neurosurg. 41 (1974), 63.
44. Russel, D. S., Rubinstein, L. J., Pathology of tumours of the nervous system. 3rd ed., p. 91. London: Arnold. 1971.
45. Sano, K., Aiba, T., Jimbo, M., Surgical treatment of cerebral aneurysms and arteriovenous malformations. Neurologica med. chir. 7 (1965), 128.
46. Serbinenko, F. A., Balloon catheterization and occlusion of major cerebral vessels. J. Neurosurg. 41 (1974), 125.
47. Sjöberg, L., Medical decision-making from a psychological point of view. Läkartidningen 73 (1976), 501.
48. Stehbens, W. E., Pathology of the cerebral blood vessels, p. 471. St. Louis, Mo.: The C. V. Mosby Co. 1972.
49. Steiner, L., Backlund, E. O., Greitz, T., Leksell, L., Norlén, G., Rähn, T., Radiosurgery in intracranial arteriovenous malformations. II. A follow-up study. International Congress Series No. 433. Neurological Surgery, p. 168 (1977).
50. Svien, H. J., McRae, J. A., Arteriovenous anomalies of the brain: fate of patients not having definite surgery. J. Neurosurg. 23 (1965), 22.
51. Troupp, H., Marttila, I., Halonen, V., Arteriovenous malformations of the brain; prognosis without operation. Acta neurochir. (Wien) 22 (1970), 125.
52. Troupp, H., Arteriovenous malformations of the brain; what are the indications for operation? Current controversies in neurosurgery, p. 210 (Morley, T. P., ed.). Philadelphia, Pa.: W. B. Saunders Company. 1976.
53. Tönnis, W., Schiefer, W., Walter, W., Signs and symptoms of supratentorial arteriovenous aneurysms. J. Neurosurg. 15 (1958), 471.
54. Tönnis, W., Symptomatologie und Klinik der supratentoriellen arteriovenösen Angiome. 1er Congrès International de Neurochirurgie, p. 205. Bruxelles. 1957.
55. Virchow, R., Die krankhaften Geschwülste, Vol. 3, p. 306. Berlin: August Hirschwald. 1863.
56. Walter, H., Die Behandlung arteriovenöser Anomalien im Gehirn mit Hilfe von Kryotherapie. Therapiewoche 22 (1972), 1542.
57. Walter, W., Bischof, W., Klinik und operative Behandlung der arteriovenösen Angiome des Stammhirns, bzw. der sogenannten Mittelhirnangiome. Neurochirurgie (Stuttgart) 9 (1966), 150.
58. Waltimo, O., The change in size of intracranial arteriovenous malformations. J. neurol. Sci. 19 (1973), 21.
59. Yaşargil, G., Microtechnical treatment of intracranial aneurysms. Microneurosurgery, p. 26 (Handa, H., ed.). Tokyo: Igaku Shoin Ltd. 1975.